Recent Results in Cancer Research 82

Fortschritte der Krebsforschung
Progrès dans les recherches sur le cancer

Editor in Chief: P. Rentchnick, Genéve
Co-editor: H. J. Senn, St. Gallen

Early Detection and Localization of Lung Tumors in High Risk Groups

Edited by P.R.Band

With 79 Figures and 66 Tables

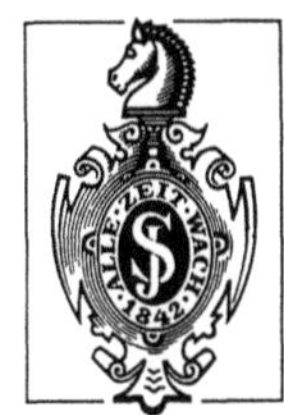

Springer-Verlag
Berlin Heidelberg New York 1982

Pierre R. Band, M.D.

Institut du Cancer de Montréal
Centre Hospitalier Notre-Dame
1560 Est, Sherbrooke
Montréal, H2L 4M1, Canada

Sponsored by the Swiss League against Cancer

ISBN-13:978-3-642-81770-0   e-ISBN-13:978-3-642-81768-7
DOI: 10.1007/978-3-642-81768-7

Library of Congress Cataloging in Publication Data. Main entry under title: Early detection and localization of lung tumors in high risk groups. (Recent results in cancer
research; v. 82) Bibliography: p. Includes index. 1. Lungs-Cancer-Diagnosis-Con-
gresses. 2. Lungs-Cancer-Congresses. I. Band, P., 1935– II. Series. [DNLM: 1. Lung
neoplasms-Diagnosis-Congresses. W1 RE106Pv. 82/WF658 E12 1981] RC280.L8E27
616.99'424075 81-21496 AACR2.

This work is subject to copyright. All rights are reserved, whether the whole or
part of the material is concerned, specifically those of translation, reprinting, re-use
of illustrations, broadcasting, reproduction by photocopying machine or similar means,
and storage in data banks. Under § 54 of the German Copyright Law where copies
are made for other than private use a fee is payable to 'Verwertungsgesellschaft Wort',
Munich.

© Springer-Verlag Berlin Heidelberg 1982
Softcover reprint of the hardcover 1st edition 1982

The use of registered names, trademarks, etc. in the publication does not imply,
even in the absence of a specific statement, that such names are exempt from the
relevant protective laws and regulations and therefore free for general use.

2125/3140–543210

Preface and Acknowledgements

Lung tumors are the leading cause of death from cancer in men, and projections indicate that within this decade the same will hold true in women. Sputum cytology provides a means to diagnose centrally located preneoplastic lung lesions and in situ carcinoma. With fluorescence bronchoscopy the possibility of localizing in situ tumors is becoming an increasing reality, whereas the chemopreventive potential of retinoids raises the hope of reversing premalignant changes.

This symposium, held on the occasion of the centennial of Notre-Dame Hospital in Montréal, addresses itself to the current status of early detection and localization procedures in groups at high risk of developing lung cancer. The conference and its publication was made possible through the generous contributions of the Exécutif du Conseil des Médecins et Dentistes de l'Hôpital Notre-Dame and La Fondation Notre-Dame; the Faculty of Medicine, the Vice-Rectorate in Research, and the Department of Continuing Medical Education of the University of Montréal; the Institut du Cancer de Montréal; the Royal College of Physicians and Surgeons of Canada; and Echanges Scientifiques Canada-France.

The financial support received from l'Association des Mines d'Amiante du Québec, la Commission des Accidents du Travail du Québec, la Fonderie CSF, Adria Laboratories of Canada Ltd., Bristol-Meyers Pharmaceutical Group, and Hoffmann-La Roche Ltd., Canada, is gratefully acknowledged.

A special debt of gratitude is owed to Miss Lynda Watson for typing all the manuscripts.

Pierre R. Band

Contents

List of Senior Authors

O.J. Balchum
Los Angeles County-University of Southern California
Medical Center, California, CA, USA

P. Band
Institut du Cancer de Montréal, Montréal, Québec, Canada

J. Chameaud
COGEMA, Service Medical du Travail, Razes, France

J. Chrétien
Hôpital Laennec, Paris, France

A. Haugen
National Cancer Institute, Bethesda, MD, USA

Y. Hayata
Tokyo Medical College, Shinjuku-ku, Tokyo, Japan

H. Kato
Tokyo Medical College Hospital, Shinjuku-ku, Tokyo, Japan

E. King
University of Alberta, Alberta, Canada

P. Kotin
Johns-Manville Corporation, Denver, CO, USA

M.L. Levin
The Johns Hopkins Medical Institutions, Baltimore, Md, USA

B. Marsh
The Johns Hopkins Hospital, Baltimore, MD, USA

N. Martini
Memorial Sloan-Kettering Cancer Center, New York, NY, USA

R. Morais
Institut de Cancer de Montréal, Montréal, Québec, Canada

M. Nasiell
Sabbatsberg Hospital, Stockholm, Sweden

G. Saccomanno
St. Mary's Hospital, Grant Junction, CO, USA

D. Sanderson
Mayo Clinic and Mayo Foundation, Rochester, MN, USA

A. Simard
Institut du Cancer de Montréal, Montréal, Québec, Canada

Carcinogenesis

Inhalation Carcinogenesis: An Overview

J. Chrétien*

Hôpital Laennec, 42 rue de Sèvres, F-75007 Paris, France

The marked rise in the incidence of respiratory carcinomas, particularly bronchogenic ones [7, 43], and the disappointing results of their treatment have led to emphasis on the importance of prevention as well as early detection. Accordingly, it is interesting to consider the pathogenesis of respiratory carcinomas and especially its relationship to inhaled substances. This contribution, from the point of view of pulmonary medicine, will first consider the environmental factors and second the specificity of the respiratory system with respect to environmental carcinogens in comparison with the other sites of tumors.

Environmental Inhaled Carcinogens

The respiratory epithelium, which consists of $60-90$ m^2 [45] of alveolar surface, conducting airway, and nasopharynx is largely and directly exposed to environmental carcinogens. A variety of environmental carcinogens (urban, domestic, and/or occupational) carried by the 12 m^3 of air normally inhaled every day can reach the respiratory epithelium. Some of these agents have been identified or suspected [7, 10, 15, 31, 34], others have not been yet recognized as oncogenic in man. These substances may act as elementary components, or they may cause complex reactions because of interactions between numerous carcinogens. The relationships may produce simple additive effects of more often synergistic effects. A complex inhaled aerosol such as tobacco smoke is especially oncogenic for the following reasons [8, 12, 13, 16]:

First, tobacco smoke aerosol contains numerous carcinogenic components with synergistic effects: Table 1 summarizes the main carcinogens that have been identified.

Second, the physical conditions of tobacco aerosol also play an important role: it is a monodispersed aerosol with a low standard deviation in the diameter of particles in suspension, and the mean size of particles is small, under 1 µm. These physical conditions favor a slow sedimentation and a prolonged stability in ambient air. This results in repetitive inhalation by smokers (and unfortunately by nonsmokers too) and after inhalation, penetration deep into the lung followed by a long retention due to the

---

* The author is indebted to Dr. R. Masse for his contributions and redaction of this paper

Table 1. Identified carcinogens in tobacco smoke (C. C. Harris, 1974)

Gas phase:
  Dimethylnitrosamine, diethylnitrosamine
  Methylethylnitrosamine, *N*-nitrosopyrrolidine
  Nitrosopiperidine

Particulate phase:
  Benzo(a)pyrene, methylbenzo(a)pyrenes
  Dibenz(a,h)acridine, dibenz(a,j)acridine
  Dibenz(c)carbazole, β-naphthylamine
  Benzo(b)fluoranthene, benzo(j)fluoranthene
  Methylfluoranthene, benzo(a)anthracene
  Chrysene, methchrysenes
  Benzo(c)phenanthrene

slow clearance from this compartment. This penetration deep into the lung is favored by the consumer himself when he voluntarily inhales the smoke deeply with each puff. If the smoker stops breathing during inspiration for one or several seconds the risk of deposition and retention of particles and gases increases even further. If we use the model drawn from the equation of Landhall (Fig. 1), we can see, for instance, that all the particles may be removed and retained in alveoli, depending on the duration of the breathhold. The slow clearance for this compartment will lead to a long contact time, in particular between the carcinogenic components and the respiratory structures.

Finally, the smoker's behavior also contributes to the pathogenicity of this carcinogen:

Inhalation is voluntary and repeated. Measures designed to protect against this will not be easily accepted. The smoker's microenvironment constantly modifies the other toxic components of his environment, for instance in occupational exposure [24]. In plastic industry workers, for example, the cloud of inhaled plastic particles, the mean size of which is usually large, only reaches the upper airway. In contrast if this same cloud passes through a burning cigarette, pyrolysis changes the size of the particles, thereby allowing them to penetrate to and be deposited in the deep regions of the lungs, and to be retained for a long time.

Although tobacco smoke is obviously the inhaled carcinogen most strongly correlated with respiratory cancers, other physical and chemical agents that act by inhalation have been detected by epidemiological and experimental studies.

Table 2 gives details of type of exposure, ways of penetration, and histological type of tumors produced. Radioactive minerals, asbestos [33, 41, 42], arsenic [23, 27], nickel [2, 18, 44], chromium [35], cadmium [5], and beryllium [30] are among the occupational factors most often incriminated.

Several other points need to be emphasized. The list of chemical environmental inhaled carcinogens is not closed. Not all the hazards have yet been recognized or clearly demonstrated, because of lack of experimental data or longitudinal epidemiological studies. Risk factors may be suddenly unmasked and become obvious, although previously unsuspected. This may happen with any material, whether introduced as a replacement (e.g., glass fiber instead of asbestos) or as a new material either in industry or in domestic environments. Hence the need to develop reliable

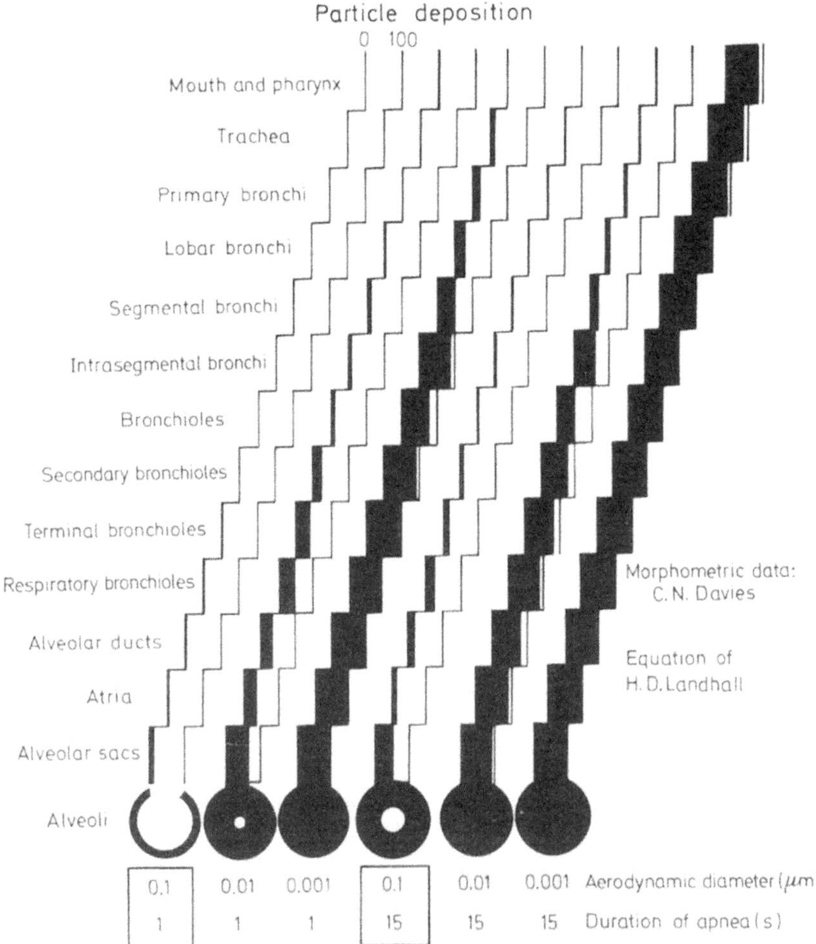

Fig. 1. Particle deposition according to aerodynamic diameter and duration of apnea

screening tests in vitro or in experimental animal models [37], such as the mutagenicity tests [1, 29] or the radon and cofactor exposure model in rats [39], to identify environmental agents that may be carcinogenic in man. Nevertheless, even by act of broad national or international agencies or laboratories, it will be difficult to solve the constantly renewed problems due to environmental agents with carcinogenic effects. Precise identification of carcinogens remains one of the major problems not yet solved in environmental pathology.

A carcinogenic effect can become suddenly obvious under the influence and by way of a cofactor, which really acts as a "revealer" (e.g., tobacco consumption in the case of asbestos or other workers). This cofactor can be a promoter or accelerator but not have its own carcinogenic effect in the sense of not being an initiating component. All the effects of environmental inhaled toxic products should be reexamined in conditions of their usual association with other components, defined as exactly as possible. Another major difficulty in assessing environmental factors concerns the risk of carcinogenicity at low doses and finally the dose-response relationship and the toxicity

Table 2. Environmental carcinogens exposure, way of penetration, and histological type of induced carcinoma

Environmental carcinogens	Type of exposure	Way of penetration	Target tissue	Carcinoma type
Virus	Environment		Various tissues	Bronchioloalveolar carcinoma among lung tumors
Physical factors				
Internal irradiation	Professional	Inhalation	Lung	Oat cell, squamous cell
External irradiation	Medical, accidental		Skin, lung	
Chemical factors				
Gas phase				
Mustard gas	Accidental	Inhalation	Lung	Oat cell
Anesthetic: Bichloromethyl ether	Professional	Inhalation	Lung	Oat cell, squamous cell
Particulate phase				
Aluminium	Professional	Oral, inhalation	Pancreas, lung, lymphoid tissues	
Beryllium	Professional	Inhalation	Lung	
Cadmium	Professional	Inhalation, skin	Lung, bladder, prostate	
Arsenic	Professional	Inhalation		Oat cell
Chromium	Professional	Inhalation	Lung	Oat cell, squamous cell adenocarcinoma
Copper	Professional	Oral, inhalation	Lung	Oat cell
Iron	Professional	Oral, inhalation	Lung	
Nickel	Professional	Inhalation	Nose	Oat cell
Lead	Environment	Inhalation		
Fibrous				
Asbestos	Professional	Inhalation	Lung, pleura, gut	Squamous cell, mesothelioma
Glass fibers	Professional environment	Inhalation	Pleura (?)	Mesothelioma (?)
Other components				
Aromatic amines	Professional, environment	Inhalation	Bladder	
Auramine	Professional	Oral, inhalation	Bladder	
Woods (dusts)	Professional	Inhalation	Pancreas, lung, lymphoid tissues	
Benzene	Professional	Oral, inhalation, skin	Bladder	
Aromatic hydrocarbons	Professional, environment	Oral, inhalation	Lung, bladder	Epidermoid
Polyvinyl chloride	Professional	Oral, inhalation	Liver, lung	Adenocarcinoma
Coal tar	Professional	Skin, inhalation	Skin, lung	
Complex aerosols				
Tobacco smoke	Environment	Oral, inhalation	Bronchial, alimentary tract, bladder	

threshold. One of the main reasons for failure of assessment by experimentation is that only one or few variables are tested and generally under conditions far from those of real human exposure.

Carcinogenic inhaled agents, regardless of their composition, lead to respiratory cancer according to local conditions and specific behavior. This explains the modalities of appearance and growth of tumors, as well as differences in individual susceptibility. On the other hand respiratory surfaces can be vulnerable not only to inhaled carcinogens, but to carcinogens entering the body by other routes. For instance, the lung can be involved in the biological chain resulting from metabolism of carcinogens brought by ingested foods and ingested or injected drugs [17]. Conversely, inhaled carcinogens can exert their effect on targets other than the lung and airways, such as tumors of the pleura in asbestos exposure or bladder or other tumors in tobacco smoke exposure.

Mechanisms Implicated in Carcinogenesis at Respiratory Surfaces: Specific and Individual Factors

For each oncogenetic process, the inhaled agents mentioned above may induce a transformation of cellular structures by interaction with macromolecules [10, 15, 22, 31, 34] according to the schema shown in Fig. 2. Many chemical oncogens form, by either spontaneous or enzymatic activation, electrophil reactants binding to cellular macromolecules. Thus, they introduce new characters in DNA or modify preexisting characters and act as derepressors of genes. This last modality is suggested for bronchoalveolar carcinoma in which viral antigens and complete virions are found in animal models and cell cultures [6, 20, 28].

If, of the inhaled oncogens, viruses, chemical carcinogens, and radioactivity have DNA as target, the target for asbestos and metals remains less definite [13, 15, 31]. There may be a relationship between the mutagenic effects of nickel and its great affinity for nucleic acids, and similarly for chromium and cobalt. For asbestos, cytogenic alterations induced by hydrocarbons absorbed on fibers have also been suggested as playing a major role, but the carcinogenicity due to asbestos fibers is obviously complex and depends partly on fiber size and type. Asbestos also acts as a cofactor, and its oncogenicity is strongly increased when associated with tobacco consumption, as shown by epidemiological studies [4, 42], and when associated with benzopyrenes, as evidenced by experimental procedures [22].

Further work is nevertheless necessary to define the mechanisms of oncogenicity of the usual chemical inhaled carcinogens and there is still a great deal of uncertainty about the precise mechanism implicated in the initiation of bronchial tumor cells. This uncertainty belongs to the "unresolved problems in carcinogenesis" discussed by Berenblum [3]. Also among the unresolved problems is that of latency time, which is correlated with the life span of each species [10] and not clearly explained by the multistage model proposed for carcinogenesis.

Besides these general concepts, which apply to all forms of carcinogenesis, cancers due to inhalation require a consideration of two other points: the specific defense mechanisms of the respiratory tract, and the reasons why the bronchial cells are usually the target for inhaled carcinogens, rather than the other cells in the lung.

The oncogenicity of inhaled carcinogens depends in large part on conditions of deposition and clearance of inhaled aerosols and is closely linked to individual factors.

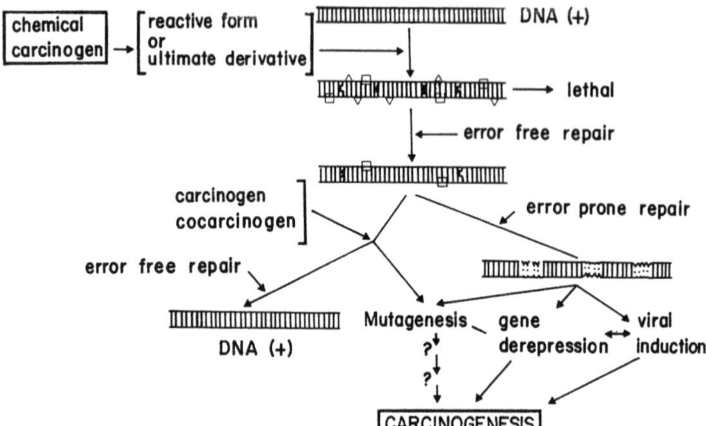

Fig. 2. Hypothetical mechanisms for chemical carcinogenesis. DNA synthesized by error prone process is indicated by the zigzag line segment. We suppose that carcinogen or cocarcinogen could also act to inhibit the error free repair process and give rise to mutagenesis [Sarasin A, Meunier-Rotival M (1976) How chemicals may induce cancer. Biomedicine 24:304–336]

The risk of cancer after inhalation of an oncogenic substance varies with the duration of contact (e.g., benzopyrene is of little oncogenicity alone, but it is highly oncogenic if given with a substance which prolongs its retention time). Thus it is of great importance to consider the specific conditions of lung clearance. This complex system includes mechanical, immunological, and biochemical factors [9, 16, 21], the study of which requires close collaboration between pneumonologists and oncologists, particularly to establish the role of specific factors and to determine individual susceptibility and risk.

In this regard various factors may be of importance, in particular genetic factors in enzymatic defenses. The Pi system could play a role in inhibiting the growth of tumor cells [19, 36], but the most important is probably the role of metabolic enzymes responsible for detoxification or activation of environmental inhaled carcinogens, such as aryl hydrocarbon hydroxylase (AHH) [11]. This substance induces less toxic molecules but also ultimately more toxic carcinogens such as 7,8-diolepoxybenzo(a)pyrene capable of linking with nucleic acid. The possibility of testing these enzymes on lymphocytes, the discovery of human groups with low, middle, or high AHH inducibility, and correlations with the presence or absence of bronchial cancers provide hope of determining individuals with a high or low risk for lung cancer [26]. Recent reports have diminished this hope [38] and additional studies are needed to assess potential susceptibility by specific analysis in the appropriate tissue, namely the respiratory epithelium.

In immunological protection, the role of alveolar macrophages in antitumor cytotoxicity, notably by the intermediary of the C3B fraction of complement, appears to be important [8, 14]. However, in a personal series [31], experimental stimulation of immunity by preventive treatment with BCG did not inhibit but rather facilitated the growth of experimental radiation-induced tumors.

Among other factors influencing susceptibility to inhaled carcinogens, hormonal, metabolic (in particular vitamin A deficiency as shown in experimental models), infectious, or toxic factors may act in a synergistic fashion [7, 10, 15, 22]. They may modify mechanical defenses such as mucociliary clearance, immunological defenses such as secretory immunoglobulins A, or respiratory epithelial components, for instance by transforming them into metaplastic cells with higher affinity for oncogenic polycyclic hydrocarbons.

Among the more than 30 types of cells that constitute the airway and alveolar structures, bronchial cells are the most vulnerable to inhaled carcinogens. The differences in renewal rate of different cells (e.g., type I pneumocytes in comparison to type II pneumocytes) and the conditions of exposure of other cells (e.g., fibroblasts in comparison to epithelial cells) could explain the difference in vulnerability. But stable aerosols including carcinogens reach and become deposited on the whole epithelium from the upper to the lower respiratory tract.

The retention of particles is prolonged deep in the lung but is much shorter in the upper respiratory tract because of mucociliary transport. However, cancers are more frequently found in main bronchi than in the lower respiratory tract and alveoli. Several hypotheses could explain this paradox of localization of cancer induced by inhaled substances [10, 15, 31]:

1) The surface area for deposition of particles in bronchi is much less than the alveolar surface. Thus, concentration of potential carcinogens is much higher. Moreover augmented deposition and stasis in different parts of the bronchial tree could occur because of local disorders of mechanical clearance: differences in regional conditions of ventilation could provoke even greater concentrations in some areas (such as the spurs or their vicinity).

2) The lung parenchyma could be quickly cleared of its particles by alveolar macrophages, whereas macrophages remain for a long time in the bronchial tree, where particles may be released. Moreover particles can directly enter and stay in bronchial cells [32].

3) Enzymes responsible for transformation of chemical inhaled carcinogens into ultimate carcinogens reside in bronchial cells.

4) Factors due to species differences about which we know little may also play a role in localization of target cells: for instance oat cell tumors arising from Kulchitsky cells are not observed in radiation-induced tumors in the rat although foci of hyperplastic cells are observed in the early stages of adenomatosis. Squamous cell carcinomas and adenocarcinomas are the usual cell types seen in these experiments.

In fact the above hypotheses do not satisfactorily explain the elective vulnerability of certain respiratory sites or cells. Why is tracheal cancer rare, compared with cancer of the proximal or distal bronchial tree? Why are the oat cell tumors of Kulchitsky cells frequent in uranium miners, even nonsmokers [40]? Why does the maximal dose to the bronchial cells not correlate with the site of radon-induced cancer [10, 15, 25, 31]? Why does asbestos exposure induce tumors from mesothelial cells in nonsmokers rather than from bronchial cells? And why does inhalation of asymmetric dimethylhydrazine induce a high rate of pulmonary angiosarcoma rather than epithelial tumors [31]?

The answers to these questions probably lie in a better knowledge of the pulmonary clearance mechanisms of each inhaled substance and their effects on cell metabolism, as well as in a better understanding of the synergistic action of carcinogens, and of the various endogenous and exogenous factors.

Specific research is needed in three fundamental areas:

1) The deposition and clearance of aerosols, especially those containing carcinogenic components, with theoretical approaches and clinical determinations in humans.
2) Specific enzymatic induction activity in the lung.
3) Specificity of the lung in immunological defense mechanisms against tumors compared to those regulating systemic defenses, and their interrelationships.

Should this ambitious program be realized, pulmonary medicine by using epidemiological and clinical data together with its specific experience in morphology, immunology, and physiology of the lung, could make a major contribution to a better approach in respiratory carcinogenesis.

References

1. Ames BN, Lee FD, Durston WE (1973) An improved bacterial test system for the detection and classification of mutagens and carcinogens. Proc Natl Acad Sci USA 70: 782–786
2. Barton RT, Hogetveix AC (1980) Nickel-related cancers of the respiratory tract. Cancer 45: 3061–3064
3. Berenblum I (1978) Established principles and unresolved problems in carcinogenesis. J Natl Cancer Inst 60: 723–726
4. Berry G, Newhouse ML, Turok M (1972) Combined effect of asbestos exposure and smoking on mortality from lung cancer in factory workers. Lancet 2: 476–479
5. Bidstrup PL, Case RA (1956) Carcinoma of the lung in workmen in the bichromates producing industry in Great Britain. Br J Ind Med 13: 260–264
6. Bucciarelli E, Ribacchi R (1972) C. type particles in primary and transplanted lung tumors induced in Balb/c mice by hydrazine sulfate: electron microscopic and immunodiffusion studies. J Natl Cancer Inst 49: 673–684
7. Chahinian AP, Chretien J (1976) Present incidence of lung cancer. Epidemiologic data and etiologic factors. In: Israel L, Chahinian AP (eds) Lung Cancer natural history, prognosis, and therapy. Academic Press, New York San Francisco London, pp 1–22
8. Chretien J (1979) Rôle du tabac dans les perturbations des défenses immunitaires pulmonaires. Rappel introductif. Nouv Presse Med 8: 2131–2134
9. Chretien J (1980) Pénétration et devenir des aérocontaminants inhalés par le poumon. In: Charpin J (ed) Allergologie. Flammarion Medecine, Paris, pp 308–323
10. Chretien J, Masse R (1976) La cancerogenèse broncho-pulmonaire. Revue des faits expérimentaux. Rev Fr Mal Respir 4: 23–45
11. Chretien J, Thieblemont M (1979) Un mécanisme intermédiaire dans la carcinogenèse pulmonaire. Nouv Presse Med 3: 1347–1350
12. Chretien J, Hirsch A, Harf A, Thieblemont M (1972) Le rôle du tabac en pathologie respiratoire. Rev Tuberc Pneumol 36: 243–280
13. Chretien J, Hirsch A, Thieblemont M (1973) Pathologie du tabac. L'expérimentation animale dans le monde. Objectifs et Méthodologie. Masson, Paris
14. Chretien J, Thieblemont M, Masse R, Chameaud J, Perraud R, Lebas F (1975) Action de la fumée de tabac sur le macrophage alvéolaire. Nouv Presse Med 32: 2327–2331
15. Chretien J, Masse R, Arnoux B, Stanislas G, Arnoux A, Queval P (1977) Agents carcinogènes et mécanismes d'action. Rev Fr Mal Respir [Suppl] 5: 19–23
16. Chretien J, Huchon G, Marsac J (to be published) Defence mechanisms of the respiratory tract. In: Freour P, Holland W (eds) Chronic non-specific respiratory disease. Henry Kimpton, London
17. Clayton DB, Shubik P (1976) The carcinogenic action of drugs. Cancer Detect Prev 1: 43–77

18. Doll R, Morgan G, Speizer FE (1970) Cancers of the lung and nasal sinuses in nickel workers. Br J Cancer 24:623−632
19. Eriksson S, Moestrup T, Hagerstrand I (1975) Liver, lung and malignant disease in heterozygous (Pi MZ) α_1-antitrypsin deficiency. Acta Med Scand 198:243−247
20. Gabelman N, Waxman S, Smith W, Douglas SD (1975) Appearance of C-type virus-like particles after cocultivation of a human tumor-cell line with rat (X.C.) cells. Int J Cancer 16:355
21. Green GM, Jakab GJ, Low RB, Davis GS (1978) Defense mechanisms of the respiratory membrane. In: Murray JJ (ed) Lung disease. State of the art. American Lung Association, New York
22. Harris CC (1974) Cause and prevention of lung cancer. Semin Oncol 1:163−166
23. Hill AB, Faning EL (1948) Studies in the incidence of cancer in a factory handling inorganic compounds of arsenic. I. Mortality experience in the factory. Br J Ind Med 5:1−15
24. Hoffmann D, Wynder EL (1976) Smoking and occupational cancers. Prev Med 5:245−261
25. James AC, Birdrall A, Greenhalg JR (1980) A model for dosimetry of the respiratory tract for inhaled radon daughters. EULEP Newsletter 21:20−21
26. Kellerman G, Shaw CR, Luyten-Kellerman M (1973) Aryl-hydrocarbon-hydroxylase inducibility and bronchogenic carcinoma. N Engl J Med 289:934
27. Lee AM, Fraumeni JF (1969) Arsenic and respiratory cancer in man: an occupational study. J Natl Cancer Inst 42:1045−1052
28. Lupulescu AP, Brinkman GL (1971) Cytoplasmic inclusion bodies in pulmonary tumors. An electron microscopic study. Amer J Clin Pathol 56:553
29. MacCann J, Choi E, Yamasaki E, Ames BN (1975) Detection of carcinogens as mutagens in the Salmonella/microsome test. Assay of 300 chemicals. Proc Natl Acad Sci USA 72:5135−5139
30. Mancuso IF (1970) Relation of duration of employment and prior respiratory illness to respiratory cancer among beryllium workers. Environ Res 3:251
31. Masse R, Arnoux B (1978) Mécanismes de la cancérisation bronchique. Rev Prat 28:4679−4685
32. Masse R, Fritsch P, Ducousso R, Lafuma J, Chretien J (1973) Rétention de particules dans les cellules bronchiques, relations possibles avec les carcinogènes inhalés. CR Acad Sci [D] (Paris) 276:2923−2925
33. McDonald AD (1976) Etudes épidémiologiques sur les maladies dues à l'amiante au Canada. Rev Fr Mal Respir [Suppl] 4:25−38
34. Miller JA (1970) Carcinogenesis by chemicals: an overview. G.H.A. Clowes memorial lecture. Cancer Res 30:559−576
35. Morgan JM (1972) Hepatic copper, manganese and chromium content in bronchogenic carcinoma. Cancer 29:710−713
36. Nash D, McLarty JW, Forston NG (1980) Pretreatment, prediagnosis immunoglobulins and alpha-1-antitrypsine levels in patients with bronchial carcinoma. J Natl Cancer Inst 64:721−724
37. NATO Advanced Research Institute. In vitro toxicity testing of environmental agents: current and future possibilities. (Abstr.) Monaco meeting, Sept 22−28, 1979
38. Paigen B, Gurtoo HL, Minowada J et al. (1977) Questionable relation of aryl-hydrocarbon-hydroxylase to lung cancer risk. N Engl J Med 297:346−350
39. Perraud R, Chameaud J, Lafuma J, Masse R, Chretien J (1972) Cancer broncho-pulmonaire experimental du rat par inhalation de radon. Comparaison avec les aspects histologiques des cancers humains. J Fr Med Chir Thorac 26:25−41
40. Saccomanno G, Archer VE, Auerbach O, Kuschner M, Saunders RP, Klein MG (1971) Histologic types of lung cancers among uranium miners. Cancer 27:515−523
41. Selikoff IJ (1976) Asbestos disease in the United States 1918−1975. Rev Fr Mal Respir [Suppl] 4:7−24

42. Selikoff IJ, Hammond EC, Churg J (1968) Asbestos exposure, smoking and neoplasia. J Am Med Assoc 204:106–112
43. Sterling TD, Pollack SV (1972) The incidence of lung cancer in the U.S. since 1955 in relation to the etiology of the disease. Am J Public Health 62:152–158
44. Sunderman FW (1976) A review of the carcinogenicities of nickel, chromium and arsenic compounds in man and animal. Prev Med 5:279–294
45. Weibel ER (1963) Morphometry of the human lung. NY Acad Press, New York

Lung Carcinogenesis During in Vivo Cigarette Smoking and Radon Daughter Exposure in Rats

J. Chameaud, R. Perraud, J. Chrétien, R. Masse, and J. Lafuma

COGEMA, Service Médical du Travail, Laboratoire de Pathologie Expérimentale, BP n° 1, F-87640 Razes, France

Introduction

The carcinogenic activity of tobacco smoke is clearly demonstrated by human epidemiologic data. Whereas in experimental animals tracheobronchial applications or injections of tars produce cancerous lesions, inhalation exposure to tobacco smoke only induces benign tumors of the bronchial epithelium and lung parenchyma [8]. The failure to induce, in animals, malignant lung tumors with inhaled cigarette smoke seems to be due to the chemical toxicity of the components of tobacco smoke. In particular, carbon monoxide and nicotine make it impossible to use the amount of inhaled smoke which would be required to induce malignant lung lesions during the relatively short life span of rodents. Since tobacco smoke is rarely inhaled alone by humans, but usually in association with other physical or chemical pollutants, we undertook experiments in which tobacco smoke was administered as a cocarcinogen to rats previously exposed to inhalations of radon and its daughter products.

During the last 10 years, we have observed the development of over 500 lung cancers in rats exposed to various cumulative doses of radon. Radon is particularly well suited for the investigation of pulmonary carcinogenic synergism because, unlike tobacco smoke and many other pollutants, it is free of chemical toxicity. Thus, experimental animals may be given within a short time period inhalations of radon at cumulative doses similar to those which induce lung cancer in humans [5, 7]. Lung cancers can be obtained in this way in rats, which almost never spontaneously develop such tumors. Further, the rate of cancer occurrence as a function of exposure is similar to that observed in epidemiologic studies of uranium miners [6, 10]. As the general condition of the animal remains good during radon exposure and during the latent period, other inhaled pollutants may be given at sublethal doses.

The cancer risk associated with tobacco smoking in the etiology of lung cancer in uranium miners is an important question [1, 3], and we undertook the investigation of the synergistic effect of cigarette smoke with radon exposure.

Materials and Methods

The inhalation exposures to radon and its daughters have been previously described by Blondeau et al. [4]. The inhalation chamber is shown in Fig. 1. For inhalation

Recent Results in Cancer Research, Vol. 82
© Springer-Verlag Berlin · Heidelberg 1982

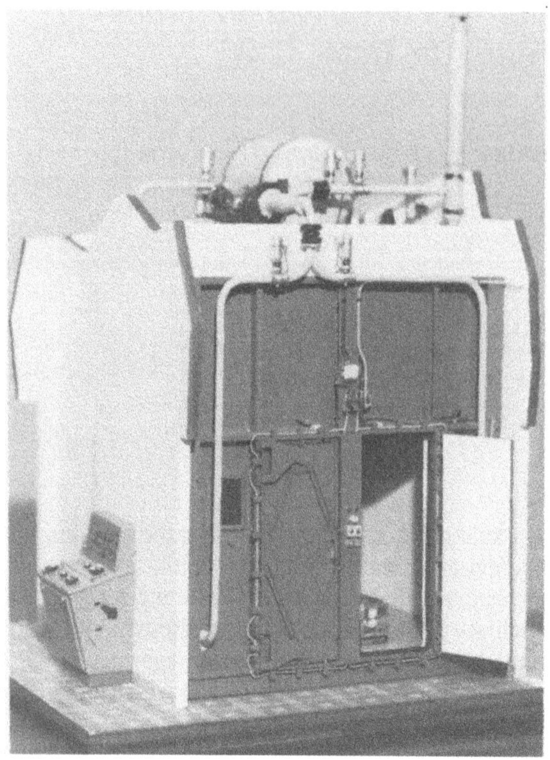

Fig. 1. Mock-up of the inhalation chamber. The source of radon-222 is radiferous lead sulfate stored in 57 containers (2 Ci per container). Radon emanations are introduced into the dilution tank located above the chamber and thoron daughters are allowed to decay for half an hour. Appropriate concentration is automatically regulated; finally the gas is introduced in two tight chambers, $10\ m^3$ each, in which 500 rats can be placed. Oxygen is provided if necessary without disturbing the equilibrium state

exposures to cigarette smoke a box, 500 l in volume, was used to expose 50 rats at a time. Cigarette smoke was produced by the simultaneous combustion of nine cigarettes (Gauloises Bleues brand). The cigarettes were placed in a cigarette holder communicating with the box. Aspiration of smoke into the chamber was ensured by means of a slight pressure differential created in the box with a vacuum pump. A ventilation system renewed the chamber atmosphere with fresh air at the end of each session of exposure to smoke.

When animals were killed, the pulmonary circulatory system of the lungs was immediately perfused in situ with physiological saline to remove blood, and the lungs were macroscopically examined for lesions.

After fixation the lungs were sectioned transversally, from above downward, in a frontal plane, into two equal parts; each part was embedded in paraffin and then cut systematically in the same direction at 20 μm thickness. The 5-μm sections selected were spread and stained with hemalum, phloxine, alcian green, and saffron.

The lung lesions were described according to the following classification derived from the TNM (tumor-node-metastasis) classification [11]:

T0	Absence of tumor	N0	No lymph node involvement
T1	Tumor < 2 mm in diameter	N1	Lymph node involvement
T2	Tumor 2−5 mm in diameter	M0	No metastasis
T3	Tumor 5−10 mm in diameter	M1	Metastasis outside the thoracic cavity
T4	Tumor > 10 mm in diameter	M2	Intrapulmonary metastases or presence of several tumors in the lungs
P0	No spread to the pleura		
P1	Spread to the pleura	M3	Association of M1 and M2

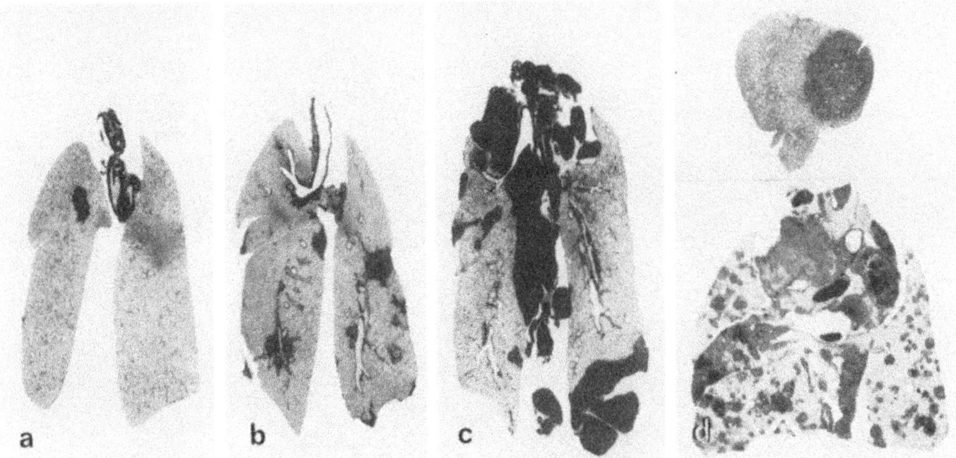

Fig. 2a–d. Staging of lung cancer. **a** T1 P0 N0 M0; **b** T2 P0 N0 M2; **c** T3 P1 N1 M3; **d** T4 P1 N1 M3 with a metastasis in the kidney; multiple nodules can be observed in the lung parenchyma, very typical of the association of radon and tobacco smoke

We thus obtained for each histological specimen a formula (e.g., T4 P1 N1 M0) used for making a simple classification and comparison. An illustration of this staging system is given in Fig. 2.

The doses of radon and its daughters chosen were 4,000, 500, and 100 work level months (WLM) because we knew from previous experiments that such doses respectively produced 30%–40%, 5%–10%, and 1%–2% lung cancers.

The smoke concentration (nine cigarettes per 500 l air) was chosen so that the animals were given 10–15 min inhalation sessions daily. The rats were exposed to smoke for 1 year, 4 days a week. Rats tolerate these exposures well, and their life span is not altered. Their lungs, loaded with tars (Fig. 3), only displayed changes in broncho-alveolar structure in the form of adenomatous metaplasia (Fig. 4), without any malignant lesion. Blood carbon monoxide levels in smoking animals were about 0.6%.

The protocol of exposure to radon and smoke is summarized in Table 1.

Results

Group 1. Two groups of 50 SPF (specific-pathogen-free) Sprague-Dawley rats distributed into cages of 10, were exposed from 3 months of age to inhalation of radon in equilibrium with its daughters at a concentration of 3,000 WL during 34 six-hour sessions, at a rate of four nocturnal sessions a week. Cumulative exposure was about 4,000 WLM. One of the groups was then exposed to smoke. The total duration of exposure to smoke under the above-described conditions was 352 h.

All rats except two smokers and three nonsmokers were examined. Histological examinations of the lung disclosed a highly significant difference between the two groups. All lungs from smokers displayed numerous lesions, often in contact with tar deposits, ranging from isolated cellular lesions to adenomatosis. Such benign lesions were much rarer in nonsmokers.

                                    J. Chameaud et al.

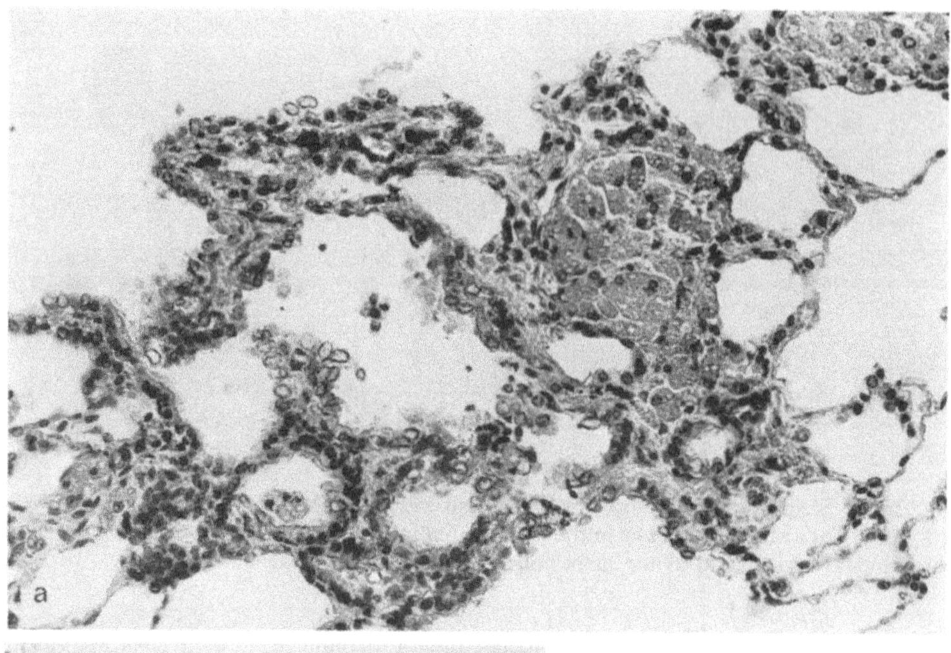

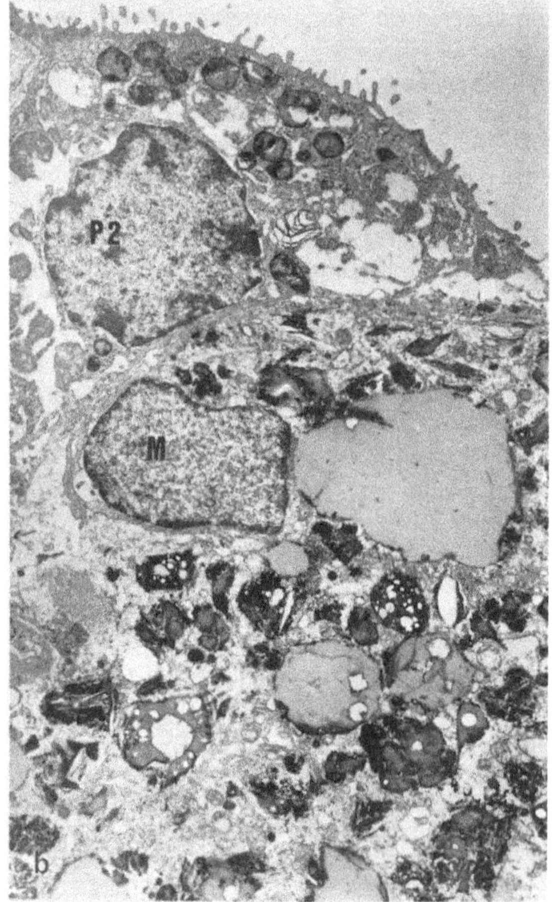

Fig. 3a, b. Legend see p 15

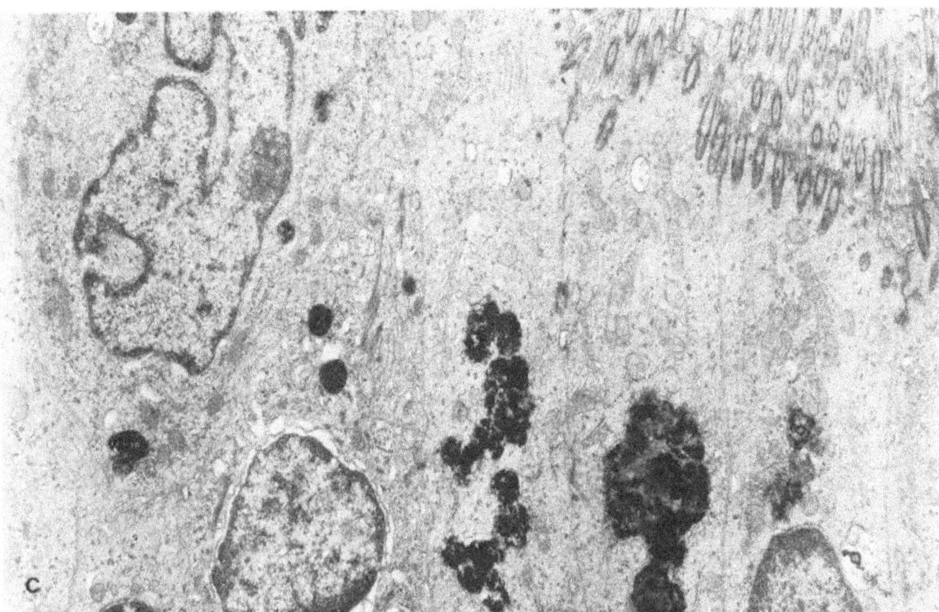

Fig. 3a–c. Lesions observed in rats from group 4. **a** Aggregated macrophages loaded with tar within an enlarged septal space surrounded by metaplastic epithelium. Hematoxylin eosin × 400. **b** Typical appearance of the dense bodies, some of them being needle shaped, due to the phagocytosis of tars by macrophages in the septum. Note the presence, on the left, of a type II pneumocytes (*P2*) with abnormal myelinic bodies (*M*). Uranyl acetate-lead × 8,000. **c** Bronchiolar epithelium storing tars in dense bodies. The storage occurs mainly in ciliated cells. Uranyl acetate-lead × 8,000

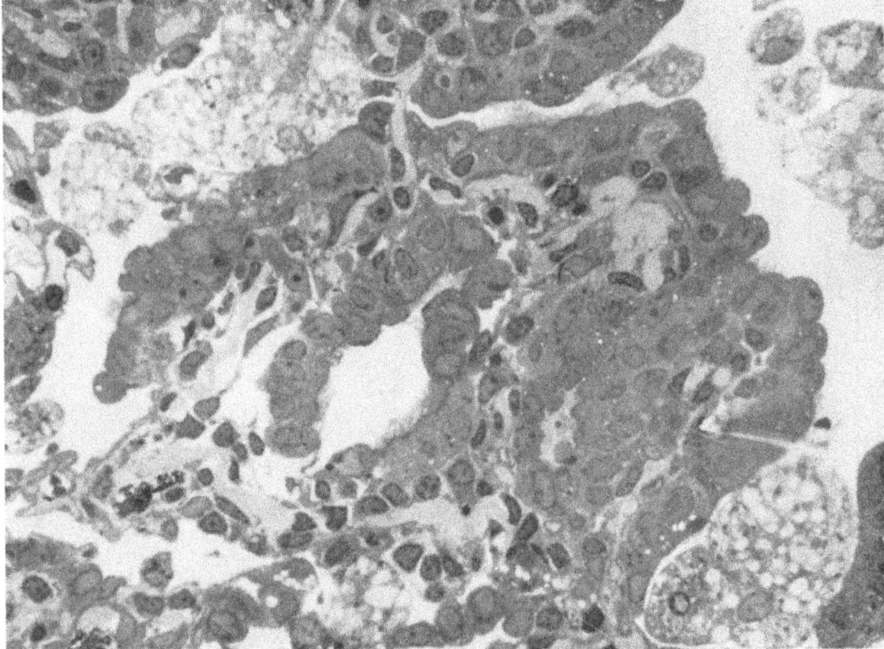

Fig. 4. Detail of focal epithelium growth around tar-loaded macrophages. Azur II × 1,200

Table 1. Protocol of exposure to radon and tobacco smoke

| Experimental group | Number of animals | Radon exposure | | | | Exposure to tobacco smoke (h) | Expected cancer incidence |
		Concentration (WL)	Cumulative dose (WLM)	Duration (weeks)	Schedule		
1	50	3,000	4,000	8	6 h per day, 4 sessions per week	0	30%−40%
	50	3,000	4,000	8		352	
2	28	3,000	500	2.5	3 h per day, 4 sessions per week	0	5%−10%
	30	3,000	500	2.5		350	
3	28	300	100	4	3 h per day, 4 sessions per week	0	1%− 2%
	30	300	100	4		350	
4	45	0	0	0	0	350	0

Table 2. Classification and number of lung cancer induced

TNM	Group 1; 4,000 WLM[a]		Group 2; 500 WLM[a]		Group 3; 100 WLM[a]		Group 4
	Radon only (50 rats)	Radon + smoke (50 rats)	Radon only (28 rats)	Radon + smoke (30 rats)	Radon only (28 rats)	Radon + smoke (30 rats)	Radon only (45 rats)
T1	2	2	2	1	0	0	0
T2	4	4	0	3	0	1	0
T3	5	6	0	2	0	0	0
T4	6	22	0	2	0	0	0
Cancer no.	17	34	2	8	0	1	0
%	34	68	7	28	0	3.3	0
P1	10	20	0	6	0	0	0
N1	1	7	0	1	0	0	0
M1	0	0	0	0	0	0	0
M2	4	16	0	1	0	0	0
M3	0	1	0	0	0	0	0

[a] Cumulative dose

Whereas in the 47 animals exposed only to radon and its daughters 17 (36%) malignant tumors were seen, such tumors occurred in 34 (71%) of the 48 rats exposed to radon and to smoke. In smokers, 62% of the tumors were T4 and 21% had lymph node metastasis (N1) as opposed to 41% and 5% respectively in nonsmokers. There was one remote metastasis (M3) in a smoker and none in nonsmokers. In addition, multiple malignant lesions (M2) were seen more frequently in smokers (35%) than in nonsmokers (9%).

Group 2. Fifty-eight rats were given a cumulative radon dose of 500 WLM in the course of 10 three-hour inhalation sessions at a concentration of 3,000 WL; 30 of these rats were also exposed to cigarette smoke for 352 h in the same way as the animals in group 1.
All lungs from smokers were examined; three of the lungs from nonsmokers could not be examined. In the smoker group nearly all animals showed isolated cellular lesion or adenomatosis, and eight cancers were seen: one T1, three T2, two T3, and two T4, with one M2. In the nonsmokers, on the other hand, there were a few benign lesions besides adenomatosis and also two cancers, both T1.

Group 3. Fifty-eight rats were given a cumulative dose of 100 WLM of radon and its daughters in the course of 17 three-hour sessions at a concentration of 300 WL. Thirty rats of this group were exposed to smoke for 352 h under the same conditions as just described. Three smoker rats were not examined. Practically all the lungs from smokers displayed isolated cellular lesions and adenomatosis, with one case of cancer (T2). The lungs from nonsmokers showed no cancer.

Group 4. Forty-five rats were given only smoke inhalations for 352 h; four rats could not be examined. No lung cancer was observed (Fig. 4). The lungs from three rats displayed adenomatosis.
The results obtained in the four experimental groups are summarized in Table 2.

Discussion

The synergistic action of cigarette smoke inhaled after exposure to cumulative doses of radon and its daughters of 4,000 WLM or of 500 WLM has been demonstrated in these two groups, since the number of cancers was significantly increased and the tumors were more invasive and metastatic. At 100 WLM we found one cancer and one suspicious adenomatosis in smokers, as opposed to none in nonsmokers, i.e., a 3%−4% incidence, whereas the expected figure was 1%−2%. The synergistic effect could not be demonstrated at this exposure level. The combined effect of cigarette smoke and radon is not additive, since cancer was not found in rats exposed only to smoke.
It will be difficult to show how this multiplicative factor varies as a function of the amount of tobacco smoked since, as the smoking level increases, a lethal threshold is rapidly reached. We do not know the number of cigarettes smoked by a human being which would be equivalent to the rat exposure. Blood carbon monoxide level in the animals during smoke exposure was 0.60%. This is the sole datum available for dosimetry comparisons together with the histopathological patterns.

The histological type of cancer was not altered by tobacco. The smoker and nonsmoker groups showed approximately 75% of epidermoid carcinoma and 20% of adenocarcinoma with a few bronchoalveolar and undifferentiated carcinomas. Interpretation derived from epidemiological surveys on the combined effects of radon and tobacco smoke are contradictory. A synergism was indicated in some studies [2, 3], but not in others [9, 12]. It has been suggested that smoking may hasten the occurrence of lung cancer in man. We have no direct evidence in rats that would substantiate the hypothesis of an effect of smoking on the latent period. However it can be observed in Table 2 that the tumors elicited in smokers are larger and more invasive. We have not observed increased mitotic indices in the tumors from smokers compared to tumors from nonsmokers. Thereby an effect of smoking on the latent period of tumors is not inconsistent. In any case, a promoting effect is the most likely mechanism involved. Indeed, in a new experiment still in progress, no potentiating effect was observed when the animals were exposed to smoke before inhaling radon. On the other hand, delayed exposure to smoke after inhalation of radon resulted in high incidence of tumors. Both features are typical of promoting agents.

Conclusion

In previous experiments covering a range of doses from 60 WLM to 12,000 WLM we have established the shape of the dose-effect relationship for radon alone. In the present experiments the carcinogenic action of tobacco smoke associated to radon was clearly demonstrated.

These studies confirm the interpretation of human epidemiological data, not only concerning uranium miners, in whom the carcinogenic factors involved are the same, but also concerning other groups at risk since, although radon exposure may play no part, smoke is always associated with other pollutants and similarly acts as a cofactor.

These results bring further evidence on the validity of our animal model which can enable us to determine the comparative toxicity of various tobaccos, the biological efficacy of various types of filters used, and more generally to investigate the cocarcinogenic effect of other physical or chemical pollutants, whether inhaled or ingested.

References

1. Archer VE, Wagoner JK, Lundin FE (1973) Lung cancer among uranium miners in the United States. Health Phys 25:351–377
2. Archer VE, Gilian JD, Wagoner JK (1976) Respiratory disease mortality among uranium miners. Ann NY Acad Sci 271:280–293
3. Band P, Feldstein M, Saccomanno G, Watson L, King G (1980) Potentiation of cigarette smoking and radiation. Evidence from a sputum cytology survey among uranium miners and controls. Cancer 45:1273–1277
4. Blondeau E, Duport P, Francois Y, Madeleine G (1973) Ensemble d'étude expérimentale du cancer pulmonaire chez le rat par irradiation. Rapp STEPPA C.E.A. France
5. Chameaud J, Perraud R, Lafuma J, Masse R (1971) Cancers du poumon expérimentaux provoqués chez le rat par des inhalations de radon. CR Acad Sci [D] (Paris) 273:2388–2389

6. Chameaud J, Perraud R, Masse R, Nenot JC, Lafuma J (1974) Lesions and lung cancers induced in rats by inhaled radon-222 at various equilibriums with radon daughters. In: Karbe E, Park JF (eds) Experimental lung cancer, carcinogenesis and bioassays. Springer, Berlin Heidelberg New York, pp 411–421
7. Chameaud J, Perraud R, Masse R, Nenot JC, Lafuma J (1976) Cancers du poumon provoqués chez le rat par le radon et ses descendants à diverses concentrations. Biological and environmental effects of low-level radiation (CR·coll Chicago, Nov 1975) II, IAEA, Vienna, pp 223–228
8. Chrétien J, Hirsch A, Thieblemont M (1973) Pathologie respiratoire du tabac. L'expérimentation animale dans le monde. Objectifs et méthodologie, Masson, Paris·
9. Cohen AF, Cohen BL (1980) Tests of the linearity assumption on the dose-effect relationship for radiation-induced cancer. Health Phys 38: 53–69
10. Perraud R, Chameaud J, Lafuma J, Masse R, Chrétien J (1972) Cancers broncho-pulmonaires expérimentaux du rat par inhalation de radon. Comparaison avec les aspects histologiques des cancers humains. J Fr Med Chir Thorac 26: 25–41
11. Renault P, Merlier M (1975) La codification T.N.M. appliquée aux cancers broncho-pulmonaires opérés. Rev Fr Mal Respir 3: 1
12. Sevc J, Kunz E, Placek V (1976) Lung cancer in uranium miners and long term exposure to radon daughter products. Health Phys 30: 433–437

Epithelial Lesions Induced by Alpha Particles and Cigarette Smoke Condensates in Organotypic Culture of Human Bronchus

R. Morais, C. Watters, A. Binda, R. Vauclair, and P. Band

Université de Montréal, Institut du Cancer de Montréal, Hôpital Notre-Dame, Départment de Biochimie, Montréal, Québec, Canada

Introduction

Epidemiological studies have established a cause and effect relationship between the increased incidence of lung cancers in miners and their exposure to radon and its daughters [1, 10, 21]. This excess in lung cancer is attributed to irradiation of the bronchial epithelium basal cells by alpha particles emitted during the radiation decay of radon gas released by uranium ore [14]. Cigarette smoking in miners has been suggested to play a role of promotion by reducing the length of the latent period [2, 20]. In experimental animals, induction of lung cancers by long-term inhalation of radon and its daughters has been demonstrated [9, 18, 19], as well as the promoting role of cigarette smoke [8].

A linear relationship has been established in humans between the incidence of lung cancer [14, 21], as well as the incidence of abnormal sputum cytology [6], and cumulative radon exposure. At cumulative radiation doses below 250 work level months (WLM), there are still considerable uncertainties regarding the somatic risks for miners exposed to alpha particles. Whether cigarette smoke could act as a promoter at these low radiation doses is also unknown. The present work has been initiated in an effort to study these problems. We report herein preliminary results obtained following the treatment of human bronchial epithelium in organ culture with low doses of alpha particles and/or cigarette smoke condensates.

Changes in Epithelium Morphology During Organ Culture of Human Bronchus

Since long-term organ culture of human bronchus has not yet been achieved routinely, it was deemed important to determine the characteristics of this biological system under our experimental conditions. Bronchial specimens from 16 cases were used in this study. All but one were males of 18−65 years of age. Lung specimens were obtained either at immediate autopsy [23] from patients with irreversible brain damage (road or work accidents) who had been kept on a respirator for $^{1}/_{2}-3$ days or at surgery from patients with lung cancer. In the latter cases, bronchi that were not grossly involved with tumor were used. It has been our experience that the morphological aspects of bronchial mucosa obtained at immediate autopsy or at surgery are essentially the same.

Recent Results in Cancer Research, Vol. 82
© Springer-Verlag Berlin · Heidelberg 1982

The experimental procedure used to culture human bronchial mucosa has been adapted from that reported by Barrett et al. [7]. Lobar and segmental bronchi were carefully dissected and small explants of $1-2$ mm^2 or larger ones of $2-3$ cm^2 were prepared and placed in 60-mm dishes with the epithelium oriented towards the gas-liquid interface. Small explants were usually covered with a coverslip. The culture medium was CMRL-1066 containing 0.1 µg hydrocortisone, 10 µg bovine insulin, and 0.1 µg β-retinyl acetate per milliliter. The medium was supplemented with 10% fetal calf serum and antibiotics. Cultures were maintained in an airtight box at 36.5° C in an atmosphere of 50% O$_2$, 45% N$_2$, and 5% CO$_2$ [7]. To ensure adequate nutrition of the explants, the medium was changed three times a week and the atmosphere reestablished.

At the time the bronchi were obtained, four major morphological traits were easily distinguishable under light microscopy. Areas of normal pseudostratified epithelium were seen (Fig. 1a), consisting of an upper layer of ciliated columnar and goblet cells and two layers of basal cells. On very rare occasions it was possible to observe areas of normal pseudostratified epithelium nearly or completely devoid of goblet cells. The human material studied revealed that this normal appearance occurred in only 26% of all the explants examined (Table 1). In fact, what was more frequently seen was basal cell hyperplasia (Fig. 1b), consisting of three or more layers of basal cells at the bottom of the epithelium, and an upper layer of ciliated columnar and goblet cells. This trait was observed in 89% of all the explants examined (Table 1). Areas of squamous metaplasia of one, two, or three layers of basal cells (Fig. 1c) were frequently seen, while partial squamous metaplasia consisting of one or more layers of basal squamous cells with a surface epithelium of ciliated cells (Fig. 1d) was observed in 11% of the explants examined (Table 1). Most of the present observations on the morphological aspects of human bronchus surface epithelium at the time of autopsy or surgery are supported by previously reported data [4, 15].

Normal pseudostratified epithelium and basal hyperplasia were the only morphological traits observed in 5% and 37% of the explants, respectively. In explants showing two or three morphological traits, the metaplastic areas covered 20% or less of the total surface area. It is worth noting that partial squamous metaplasia was always found associated with basal hyperplasia and squamous metaplasia.

The major morphological traits identified at the time of autopsy and surgery in human specimens were maintained for up to 35 days (Table 2). In addition, areas of regeneration of the epithelium (Fig. 1e) were found at day 14 in most of the explants examined and persisted up to 35 days in some of them.

In areas of normal pseudostratified epithelium and basal cell hyperplasia, goblet cells decreased in number and were rarely seen at the end of the culture period. On the other hand, all explants examined at day 14 showed areas of squamous metaplasia which increased as a function of time and usually represented, on day 35, more than

---

Fig. 1a–e. Morphological aspects of the surface epithelium of human bronchi obtained either at ▶ immediate autopsy or at surgery. **a** Normal pseudostratified columnar epithelium with goblet cells, ciliated cells, and basal cells. **b** Basal cell hyperplasia with two or more layers of basal cells at the bottom of the epithelium and an upper layer of ciliated columnar and goblet cells. **c** Squamous metaplasia with atrophy. **d** Partial squamous metaplasia with layers of basal cells and a surface epithelium of ciliated cells. **e** Area of regeneration of the surface epithelium (14-day culture). Hematoxylin-saffron-phloxine × 400

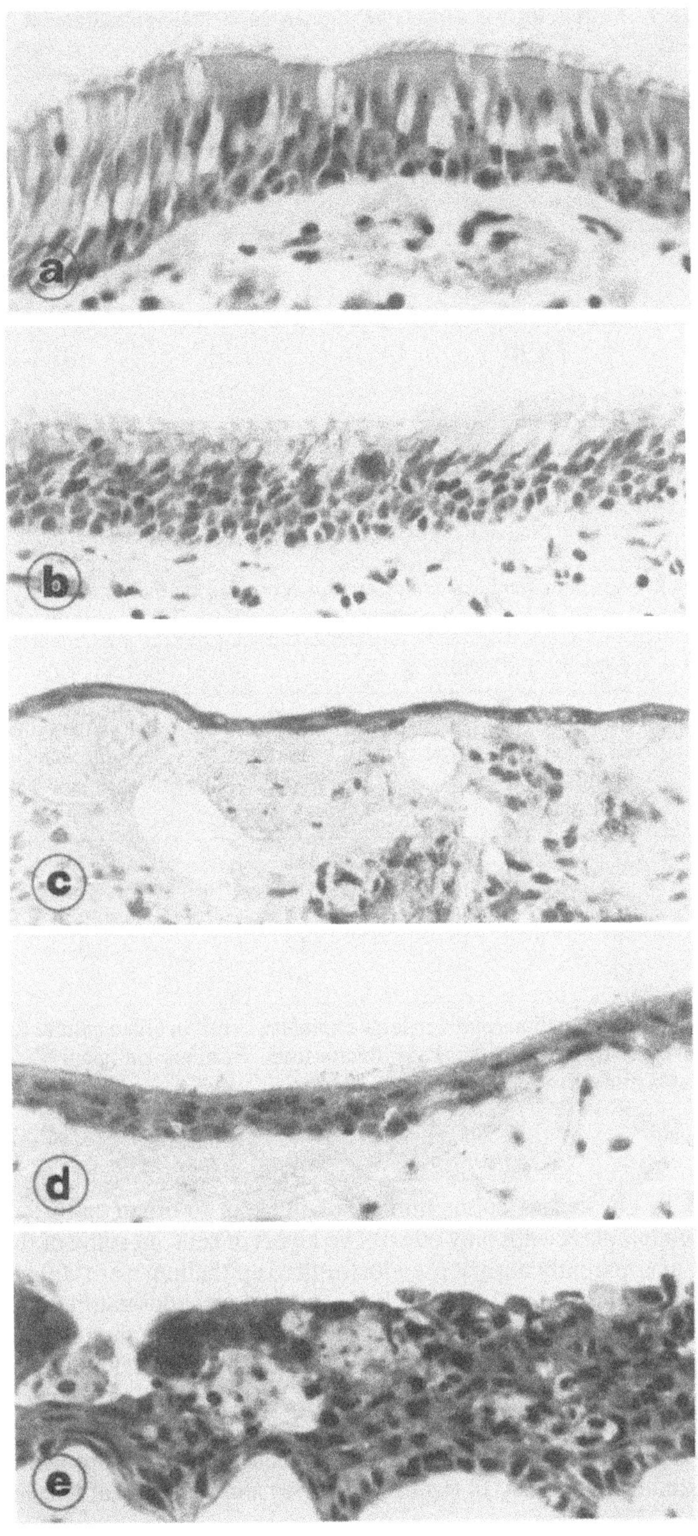

Table 1. Morphological aspects of human bronchial epithelium at immediate autopsy or surgery

Explants (%) showing				
Pseudostratified epithelium (normal)	Basal cell hyperplasia	Partial squamous metaplasia	Squamous metaplasia	Regeneration of the epithelium
[A]	[B]	[C]	[D]	[E]
26	89	11	42	0

[A]	[A, B]	[A, D]	[B]	[B, D]	[B, C, D]
5	16	5	37	26	11

Three different sections of 25 large explants (1 cm^2) were examined under the light microscope. Sections on glass slides were stained with hematoxylin saffron phloxine

Table 2. Morphological aspects of human bronchial epithelium as a function of time in organ culture

Day	Explants (%) showing				
	Pseudo-stratified epithelium (normal)	Basal cell hyperplasia	Partial squamous metaplasia	Squamous metaplasia	Regeneration of the epithelium
0	26	89	11	42	0
7	0	17	17	83	0
14	20	0	20	100	80
21	0	17	17	100	33
35	17	17	67	83	17

Three different sections of seven large explants (1 cm^2) in organ culture for 7, 14, 21, and 35 days were examined under the light microscope. Sections on glass slides were stained with hematoxylin-saffron-phloxine

80% of the surface epithelium. Explants kept in organ culture for at least 2 months were metaplasic with only one or two layers of cells. In some of the explants, however, foci of apparently normal pseudostratified epithelium were still found. Associated to a tendency towards a change from normal pseudostratified epithelium and basal hyperplasia to squamous metaplasia was a decrease in the thickness of the epithelium, which attained a minimum by about day 14 (from 32 ± 9 μm at the time of autopsy or surgery to 10 ± 5 μm) and stayed at that level for at least 30 more days. Concomitantly with the development of areas of regeneration of the epithelium, the percentage of ^{3}H-thymidine labeled surface epithelial cells on human bronchial explants attained a maximal value at day 14 (from 7%−14%) and persisted at that level for 15 more days before decreasing.

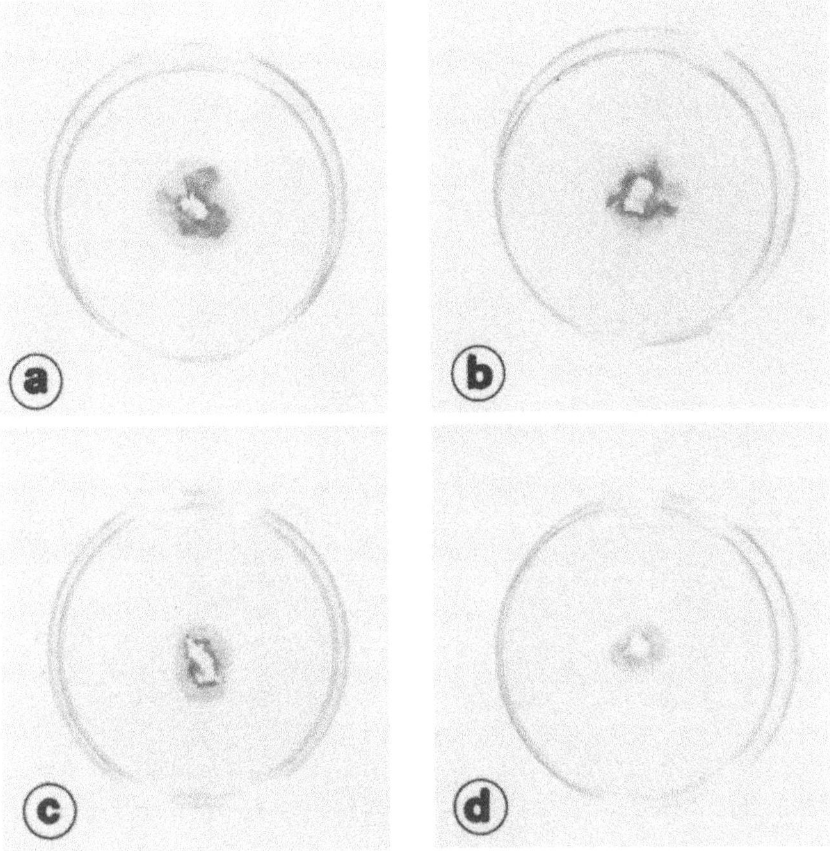

Fig. 2a–d. Outgrowths of cells from bronchial explants maintained for 21 days in organ culture. Outgrowths were stained with Giemsa. The clear areas at the center of the outgrowths were occupied by the explants. Epithelial cells with a polygonal shape were usually found in darkly stained areas and large flat cells in weakly stained ones. **a** Control explant. **b** Explants treated with alpha particles (2 rad/day). **c** Explants treated with 50 µg CSC/ml. **d** Explants treated with alpha particles and CSC

Outgrowth of Epithelial Cells from Explant Tissues

Cells grew out onto the surface of the dishes within 3 days, when pieces of bronchial epithelium were explanted into culture dishes. The area occupied by the outgrowths reached a maximum by about 3–4 weeks (Fig. 2a). Cellular sheets usually sloughed off the substratum 3–4 weeks later. When the explants were transferred into other dishes, new outgrowths of about the same surface areas were generated within 3 weeks. Explants can be transferred and can generate outgrowths at least four times. When explants are removed, however, cellular sheets slough into the medium 3–5 days later. Similar observations have been reported recently [11, 12, 22].

Epithelial cells with a polygonal shape (Fig. 3a) accounted usually for 50%–90% of the outgrowth surface area. The remaining area was occupied by large, spread-out cells (Fig. 3b) which stained more weakly with Giemsa than the polygonal cells

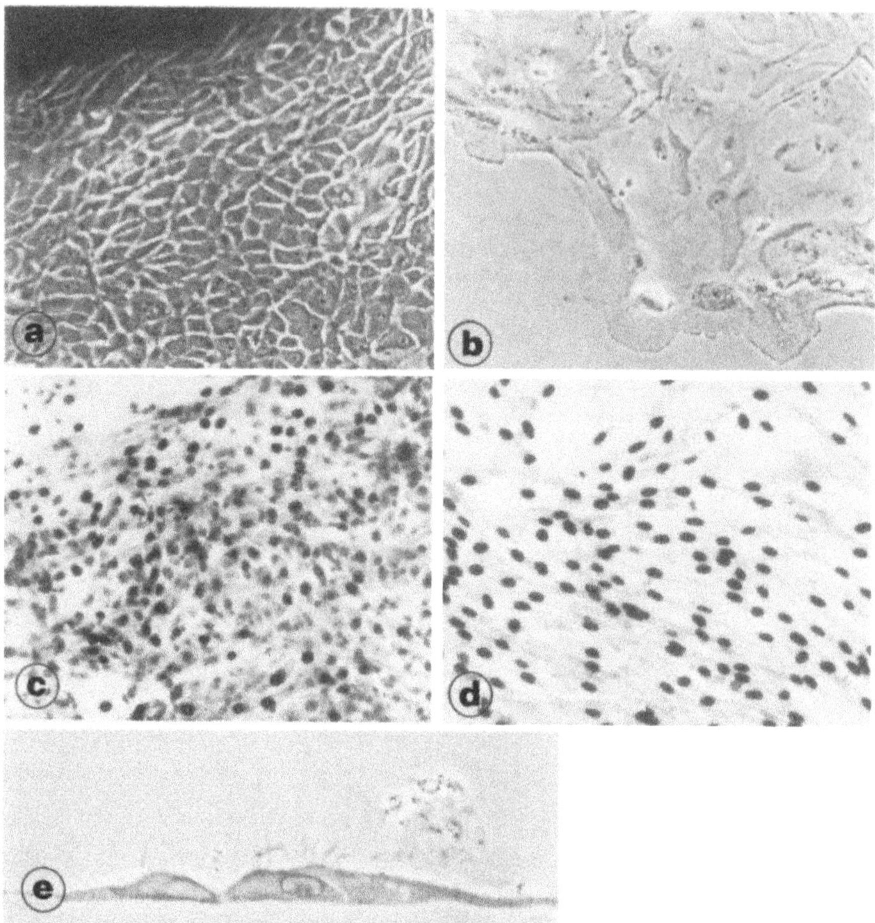

Fig. 3a—e. Morphological aspects and ^{3}H-thymidine labeling of cells in outgrowths. **a** Polygonal epithelial cells in a 21-day outgrowth. The dark area in the upper left corner is a portion of the explant. Living. Phase contrast × 100. **b** Large, flat cells at the periphery of a 21-day outgrowth. Living. Phase contrast × 100. **c** Polygonal cells labeled with ^{3}H-thymidine in a 14-day outgrowth. Phase contrast × 100. **d** ^{3}H-Thymidine labeling of fibroblasts. Phase contrast × 100. **e** Cross section of epithelial cells with cilia. Cloudlike material pushed away by cilia is also seen. Phase contrast ×1,000

(Fig. 2a). At day 14, most of the epithelial cells around the explants were incorporating ^{3}H-thymidine (Fig. 3c). At 3−4 weeks of culture, when the outgrowths attained their maximal surface area, some rare cells were still able to incorporate ^{3}H-thymidine. In about 20% of the outgrowths examined, areas of fibroblasts with a high labeling index were seen (Fig. 3d). Ciliary activity was observed in a small proportion of the polygonal cells (Fig. 3e), suggesting that differentiation continued to occur in culture.

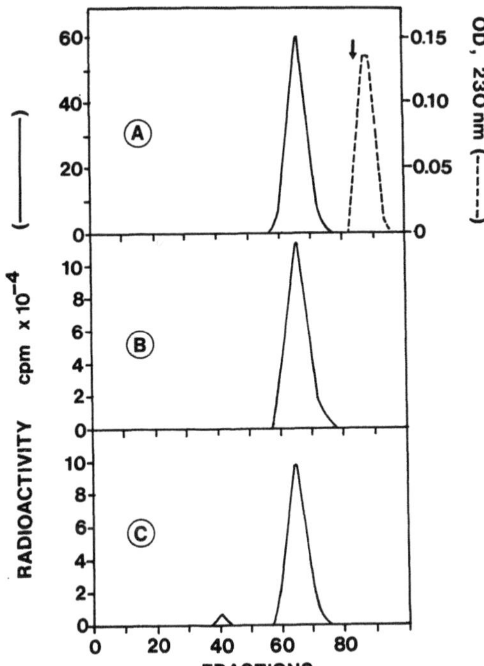

Fig. 4A–C. Isolation and stability of the complex DTPA-[241]Am. Americium nitrate was complexed to DTPA (10^{-2} M) in HCl 1.0 N. **A** Complex was separated from excess DTPA [13] on Sephadex G-25 with NaCl 0.15 M as eluant. Arrow indicates the elution fraction of [241]Am alone. **B** Complex kept at room temperature for 6 months. **C** Complex added to culture medium and incubated at 36.5° C for 3 days

Effect of Alpha Particles and Cigarette Smoke Condensates on Human Bronchus in Organ Culture

As a source of alpha particles, we resorted to the use of americium ([241]Am), an actinide with an alpha energy of 5.5 MeV. Americium was complexed to the chelator diethylenetriamine pentaacetic acid (DTPA), which is used as a therapeutic agent to remove [241]Am in experimental animals [16] or in man in case of accidental contamination with actinides [5, 17]. The complex prepared in acid solution [13] was fractionated from excess DTPA on Sephadex G-25 (Fig. 4a). Once prepared, the complex was stable for several months at room temperature (Fig. 4b) or for 3 days when incubated at 36.5° C in the culture medium (Fig. 4c). In the latter case, some of the complex became absorbed to high molecular weight components present in fetal calf serum and was eluted in the void volume. Cigarette smoke condensates (CSC) in acetone were a generous gift from Dr. Y. Chouroulinkov (Villejuif, France).

Large explants were kept in organ culture for 14 days, the time when labeling index attained its maximal value, and were cut into pieces of about 0.5 cm² and transferred into other dishes. Microscopic examination of sections of these explants revealed the presence of the major morphological traits previously described. Small explants of 1–2 mm² that had generated outgrowths during the 14-day period were also transferred into other dishes. Explants were treated as a function of time with either DTPA-[241]Am, or CSC, or DTPA-[241]Am plus CSC. At the end of the treatment, some of the explants were implanted into nude mice (Swiss, NIH, Bethesda) and the other explants processed for autoradiography and histology. Explants chosen at random were treated with 2 rad [241]Am per day and/or 50 µg CSC/ml for 28 days. Higher doses of alpha particles and CSC were found to elicit in a few days the degeneration of the

                                                                  R. Morais et al.

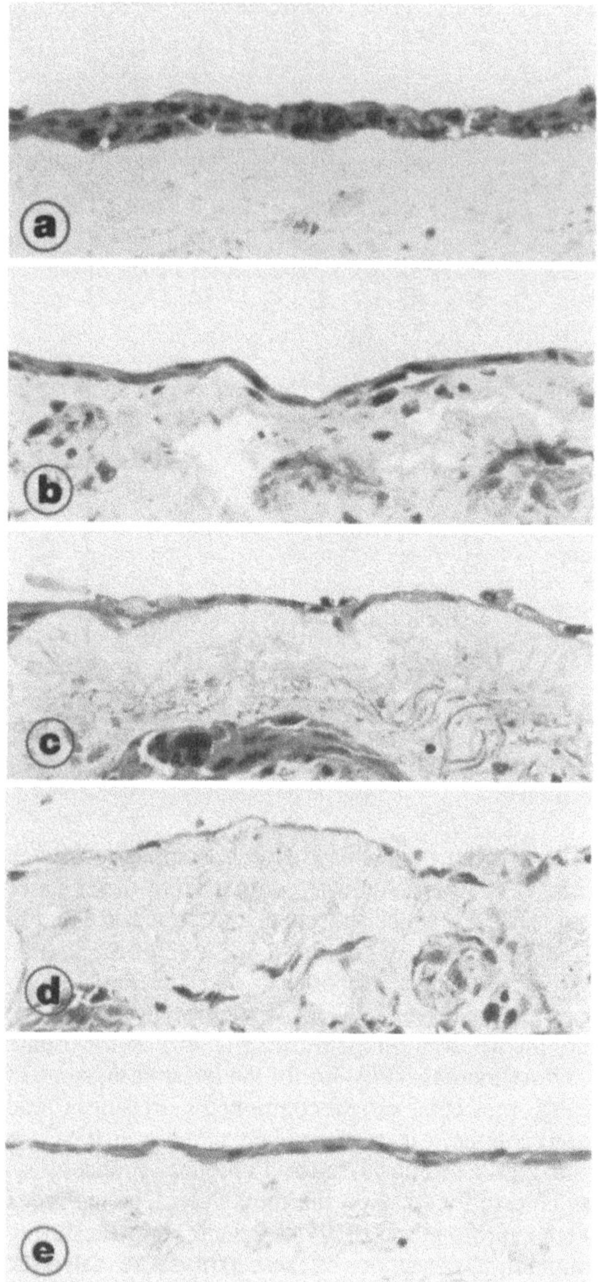

Fig. 5a–e. Morphological aspects of the surface epithelium of human bronchi treated with alpha particles and CSC. Squamous metaplasia in explants treated with: **a** Alpha particles for 14 days; **b** Alpha particles for 28 days; **c** CSC for 21 days; **d** CSC for 28 days. Hematoxylin-saffron-phloxine × 400

surface epithelium and to prevent the formation of outgrowths. Control experiments demonstrated that DTPA (10^{-9} M) and acetone (0.05%) did not alter the morphological appearance of the surface epithelium, the total surface area, or the type of cells in outgrowths.

Reduced areas of normal pseudostratified epithelium, basal hyperplasia, and partial squamous metaplasia were seen in all explants treated with alpha particles and/or CSC

Table 3. Surface area of outgrowths following treatment with cigarette smoke condensate or radioactivity or both (3 weeks' treatment)

Treatment		Area (mm^2) $\pm$ SD (N)	Range
CSC (μg/ml)	DTPA-^{241}Am (rad/day)		
0	0	220 $\pm$ 67 (6)	116–308
0	2	74 $\pm$ 24 (6)	39–100
50	0	37 $\pm$ 16 (6)	11– 52
50	2	24 $\pm$ 16 (6)	0– 52
Before treatment (2 weeks)		94 $\pm$ 32 (30)	40–165

for 7 days. A week later, the only morphological trait observed in all explants treated with alpha particles (Fig. 5a) was squamous metaplasia consisting of one, two, or three layers of cells. Foci of epithelium regeneration were sometimes seen in some of the explants treated with alpha particles, but they were not seen in explants treated with CSC. After 4 weeks of treatment with alpha particles, the epithelium was atrophic and consisted of a single layer of flattened cells (Fig. 5b). Some of these cells were still able to incorporate ^{3}H-thymidine. Atrophic squamous metaplasia of one and sometimes two layers of cells was detected at day 21 in explants treated with CSC (Fig. 5c). The surface epithelium had disappeared by day 28 (Fig. 5d) but not the glandular epithelium, which still appeared to be intact. In the presence of DTPA-^{241}Am plus CSC, atrophic squamous metaplasia was observed at day 14 (Fig. 5e) and the surface epithelium had degenerated by day 21.

The inhibitory effect demonstrated by alpha particles and CSC on the proliferation and differentiation of the surface epithelial cells was also observed in outgrowths. At day 14, when explants were transferred into other dishes, the mean surface area of outgrowths was 94 mm^2 (Table 3). Three weeks later, control explants generated outgrowths with a mean surface area of 220 mm^2. Outgrowths generated by explants treated with alpha particles and CSC had a mean surface area reduced by more than 60% and 80%, respectively. In the presence of DTPA-^{241}Am plus CSC, the mean surface area was further reduced, although not statistically significantly more than with CSC alone. As compared to controls, the surface area of epithelial cells with a polygonal shape (moderately stained with Giemsa) was reduced in outgrowths generated by explants treated with alpha particles or CSC (Fig. 2b, c). A narrow layer of epithelial cells was seen under the light microscope at the periphery of explants treated with alpha particles plus CSC (Fig. 2d). The mean surface area of outgrowths was mainly accounted for by large flat cells weakly stained with Giemsa. Epithelial cells with ciliary activity were still seen, however, in explants examined.

Explants treated with alpha particles and/or CSC for 2–4 weeks were implanted into nude mice. Explants examined 6 months later revealed a normal-like pseudostratified surface epithelium, and no preneoplastic or neoplastic lesions were detected as late as 1 year later.

Conclusion

Alpha particles and cigarette smoke have been shown to cause cancer in humans and in experimental animals. The present study illustrates the potential for using human bronchi in organ culture for the study of the effects of these carcinogenic agents. They induce squamous metaplastic changes, alterations that are regarded as potentially preneoplastic events. Such changes have been shown to occur far more frequently in cigarette smokers than in nonsmokers [3, 4] and sputum cytology studies of uranium workers revealed that the frequency of abnormal cytology was significantly dependent on the duration of uranium mining and of cigarette smoking [6]. Work is in progress to study the effect of fractionated low doses of radiation on the surface epithelium of explants treated or not with CSC, and their potential to generate new outgrowths as a function of time. Considering that progression from initiation to invasive epithelial cancer may often take up to 20 years or more in man, it is hoped in this way to detect in a relatively short time preneoplastic and neoplastic lesions induced by these or other carcinogenic agents.

Acknowledgments. This work was supported by a grant from Health and Welfare, Canada. R. M. is a Chercheur-Boursier from Le Conseil de la Recherche en Santé du Québec. A. B. is recipient of a studentship from Le Ministère de l'Education du Québec. We thank Dr. René Béique for helpful discussions and Mrs. France Lafontaine for typing the manuscript.

References

1. Archer VE, Wagoner JK (1973) Lung cancer among uranium miners in the United States. Health Phys 25: 351–371
2. Archer VE, Wagoner JK, Hyg SD, Lundin FE (1967) Uranium mining and cigarette smoking effects on man. Environ Res 1: 370–383
3. Auerbach O, Stout AP, Hammond EC et al. (1961) Changes in bronchial epithelium in relation to cigarette smoking and in relation to lung cancer. N Engl J Med 265: 253–367
4. Auerbach O, Hammond EC, Garfinkel L (1979) Changes in bronchial epithelium in relation to cigarette smoking. N Engl J Med 300: 381–386
5. Bair WJ, Trombopoulous EG, Park JF (1962) Distribution and removal of transuranic elements and cerium deposited by the inhalation route. In: Diagnosis and treatment of radioactive poisoning. IAEA and WHO, Vienna, p 319
6. Band P, Feldstein M, Saccomanno G, Watson L, King G (1980) Potentiation of cigarette smoking and radiation. Evidence from a sputum cytology survey among uranium miners and controls. Cancer 45: 1273–1277
7. Barrett LA, McDowell EM, Frank AL, Harris CC, Trump BF (1976) Long-term organ culture of human bronchial epithelium. Cancer Res 36: 1003–1010
8. Chameaud J, Perraud R, Chrétien J, Masse R, Lafuma J (1979) Experimental study of the combined effects of inhalation of radon daughter products and tobacco smoke. In: 19th annual Hanford life sciences symposium on pulmonary toxicology of respirable particles. Richland, USA
9. Chameaud J, Perraud R, Lafuma J, Masse R, Pradel J (1979) Lesions and lung cancer induced in rats by inhaled Radon^{222} at various equilibriums with radon daughters. In: Karbe E, Parke JP (eds) Experimental lung cancer carcinogenesis. Springer, Berlin Heidelberg New York, p 411
10. De Villiers AJ, Windisch JP (1964) Lung cancer in a fluorspar mining community. 1. Radiation, dust, and mortality experience. Br J Ind Med 21: 94–109
11. Jechner JF, Haugen A, McClendon IA, Pettis EW, Trump BF, Harris CC (1980) Clonal growth requirements and serial culture of adult human bronchial epithelium. J Cell Biol 87: 231a

12. Kato Y, Stoner GD, McIntire KR et al. (1979) Immunological markers of human bronchial epithelial cells in tissue sections and in culture. J Natl Cancer Inst 62: 1177–1185
13. Lafuma J, Nenot JC, Morin M (1968) Méthode nouvelle d'étude de l'efficacité des chelateurs de la série des acides polyamines pour la décontamination interne. Rapport CEA-R-3519, Commissariat à l'énergie atomique, France
14. Lundin FE, Wagoner JK, Archer VE (1971) Radon daughter exposure and respiratory cancer: quantitative and temporal aspects. NIOSH and NIEHS joint monograph 1. National Technical Information Service, Springfield, VA
15. McDowell EM, Barrett LA, Glavin F, Harris CC, Trump BF (1978) The respiratory epithelium. I. Human bronchus. J Natl Cancer Inst 61: 539–549
16. Nenot JC, Morin M, Skupinski W, Lafuma J (1972) Experimental removal of ^{144}Ce, ^{241}Am, ^{242}Cm and ^{238}Pa from the rat skeleton. Health Phys 23: 635–640
17. Norwood WD (1962) Removal of plutonium and other transuranic elements from man. In: Diagnosis and treatment of radioactive poisoning. IAEA and WHO, Vienna, p 307
18. Perraud R, Chameaud J, Masse R, Lafuma J (1970) Cancers pulmonaires expérimentaux chez le rat après inhalation de radon associé à des poussières non radioactives. CR Acad Sci [D] (Paris) 270: 2544–2545
19. Perraud R, Chameaud J, Lafuma J, Masse R, Chrétien J (1972) Cancer bronchopulmonaire expérimental du rat par inhalation de radon. Comparaison avec les aspects histologiques des cancers humains. J Fr Med Chir Thorac 26: 25–41
20. Saccomanno G, Archer VE, Auerbach O, Saunders RP, Brennan LM (1974) Development of carcinoma of the lung as reflected in exfoliated cells. Cancer 33: 256–269
21. Sevc J, Kunz E, Placek V (1976) Lung cancer in uranium miners and long-term exposure to radon daughter products. Health Phys 30: 433–437
22. Stoner GD, Harris CC, Myers GA, Trump BF, Connor RD (1980) Putrescine stimulates growth of human bronchial epithelial cells in primary culture. In Vitro 16: 399–406
23. Trump BF, Valigorsky JM, Dees JH et al. (1974) Cellular change in human disease. A new method of pathological analysis. Hum Pathol 4: 89–109

Asbestos Carcinogenesis:
Asbestos Interactions and Epithelial Lesions
*in Cultured Human Tracheobronchial Tissues and Cells**

A. Haugen and C. Harris**

National Cancer Institute, National Institutes of Health, Human Tissue Studies Section, Laboratory of Experimental Pathology, Division of Cancer Cause and Prevention, Bethesda, MD, USA

Introduction

Asbestos, the commercial name of minerals that form fibers when crushed, occurs as two groups called serpentine and amphibole. Chrysotile is the fibrous form of serpentine and this white asbestos accounts for over 90% of the world's usage. Crocidolite, amosite, and anthophyllite are widely used amphiboles. These fibrous varieties are different in both physical and chemical characteristics [13].
Asbestos causes several diseases such as asbestosis, bronchial carcinomas, and both pleural and peritoneal mesotheliomas [13]. The association between asbestos inhalation and lung disease has been recognized for many years. In 1935, Lynch and Smith [26] suggested the association between asbestos exposure and lung cancer, an uncommon disease at that time. Since then asbestos has continued to attract attention as an occupational and public health hazard.
Asbestos fibers are the major cause of mesothelioma. A positive association between occupational exposure to asbestos and risk of bronchogenic carcinoma was first established by Doll [6]. Epidemiological studies found an increased incidence of bronchogenic carcinoma in workmen exposed to asbestos fibers. Although commercial forms of asbestos have been shown to be oncogenic [32], the carcinogenic potency of the different types is still debated. The prevalence of asbestos-related lung disease has been studied extensively among insulators, shipyard workers, and asbestos miners [42]. However, since asbestos is a component of many materials, exposure to asbestos in the general workplace is widespread. High exposure level to asbestos for brief periods of time, e.g., a month, can cause cancer 15–20 years later. Even extremely low levels of asbestos exposure may have a carcinogenic effect [15, 28, 52]. The combination of cigarette smoking with exposure to asbestos increases the risk of bronchial cancer; 90% of the asbestos-related cancers are a result of its combined effect with cigarette smoke, while asbestos caused only a limited increase in carcinoma in nonsmokers [40]. In contrast, no relationship has been demonstrated between tobacco smoking and the incidence of mesothelioma [11]. Asbestos is both a

---

* Guest worker sponsored in part by the Norwegian Council for Scientific and Industrial Research and Research Fellowship awarded by NATO
** The authors would like to thank Dr. U. Saffiotti for valuable comments and Mrs. S. Dorman for her secretarial assistance

cocarcinogenic and a carcinogenic agent in the etiology of bronchogenic carcinoma [2, 8, 39, 40]. The most common types of bronchogenic cancer are adenocarcinoma and squamous cell carcinoma [53]. Epidemiological studies have shown that asbestos workers may also expect a higher morbidity from cancer at other sites, for example, stomach and intestine [21, 41].

Asbestos is in widespread use in hundreds of products [16]. Several investigators have reported finding asbestos bodies (ferruginous bodies) in lung tissue from persons with no known occupational exposure to asbestos dust [5]. Owing to its contamination of both the workplace and the general environment, asbestos is considered to be one of the leading public health concerns of our time. The study of cellular reactions and damage in the lung caused by asbestos fibers is therefore of special importance.

Experimental Studies Relevant to the Evaluation of Carcinogenic Risk of Asbestos in Respiratory Tract

Animal Studies

The most realistic route of asbestos administration to animals is by inhalation. Intratracheal instillation may also be quite relevant to study the pathogenesis of the respiratory tract. The major pathological effects caused by asbestos are fibrogenesis and carcinogenesis. A study of biological properties of asbestos is experimentally difficult owing to both the variable contamination of asbestos by other minerals and the variation in size distribution of the fibers.

In 1941, Nordmann and Sorge [34] found lung tumors in mice exposed to asbestos dust, but found only two bronchogenic carcinomas in 10 mice. Later Lynch et al. [27], did similar experiments, but they were unable to demonstrate any proof of the carcinogenicity of asbestos fibers. Reeves et al. [36, 37], found squamous carcinomas of the lung in rats after inhalation of crocidolite, chrysotile, or amosite for 2 years with a total exposure time of about 1,500 h. These effects were ascribed by the authors to increased amounts of trace metals from the worn hammer of the mill used to produce the asbestos fibers. After a short period of either chrysotile or crocidolite inhalation, guinea pigs demonstrated increased cellular proliferation and hyperplasia of bronchial epithelium [3, 17]. Gross and his collaborators [10] found lung cancer in 30% of the rats surviving 16 months after inhalation exposure to chrysotile. More recently, Wagner et al. [51] reported a study where rats were exposed by inhalation to five types of asbestos, each for periods up to 24 months. Wistar rats were exposed to dust clouds of the UICC standard reference samples for different time periods from 1 day to 2 years. Lung cancers were produced by all samples and a positive association between asbestosis and tumor incidence was demonstrated. Lung cancers were observed in 247 of the 713 rats exposed to asbestos fibers. These experimental studies demonstrate clearly the carcinogenicity of asbestos.

The cocarcinogenic effect of chrysotile fibers was recently investigated by Topping and Nettesheim [48]. Using rat tracheal transplants preexposed to a nondetectable tumorigenic dose of 7,12-dimethylbenz[a]anthracene, enhancement of the tumor response was observed following exposure to 200 µg chrysotile. These results suggest that chrysotile can act as a cocarcinogen in this animal model. Chrysotile has also been shown to be weakly carcinogenic in rat tracheal transplants [49].

There are two properties of asbestos fibers that need to be considered as potentially carcinogenic. First, the chemical composition, including trace metal content or the presence of hydrocarbon or other organic contaminants, may play a major role in the etiology of bronchogenic carcinomas. Second, the physical structure of asbestos fibers influences the carcinogenic potential. Supporting evidence for the physical factor hypothesis is stronger when one considers mesotheliomas caused by asbestos. For example, brucite, fine fiberglass, glass powder, and aluminium oxide fibers as well as all types of asbestos [44, 50] induce mesotheliomas with approximately equal efficiency provided that the fibers or particles are in the right size range (greater than 8 μm in length and less than 1.5 μm in diameter), indicating that chemical properties of the fibers are unlikely to be the main factor producing mesotheliomas. The report by Wagner et al. [51], also supports this interpretation. They demonstrated that benzene-extracted crocidolite produced the same number of tumors as did nonextracted crocidolite. Gross [9] considers fibers shorter than 5 μm to have little or no carcinogenic effect in the pulmonary tree. However, further studies are needed to substantiate this conclusion. When one considers the epidemiological evidence relating physical characteristics of fibers and their oncogenic potential, there is no evidence that glass fibers cause tumors in humans [1, 7]; however, long fibers with a diameter of 1 μm or less have been produced in large scale for only a relatively short time, i.e., approximately 10 years. Since the latency period for lung cancers is generally 2–3 decades, epidemiological data in the future may permit different conclusions. Results from an initial analysis of data from 13 factories in Europe are expected in 1981 [20].

Asbestos fibers contain metals including iron, magnesium, and aluminium as major constituents and nickel, chromium, cobalt, and others as trace elements. Nickel and chromium are considered to be respiratory carcinogens [46]. Asbestos fibers may, because of their adsorptive capacity, act in conjunction with metals and chemical carcinogens. Experimental carcinogenesis studies in animal models using different types of asbestos fibers and benzo[a]pyrene have shown clearly that exposure to chrysotile and benzo[a]pyrene enhances the carcinogenicity of the benzo[a]pyrene [35]. Using model systems [22], Lakowicz and Hylden demonstrated that benzo[a]pyrene adsorbed to mineral particulates resulted in more rapid transportation into membranes than microcrystals of benzo[a]pyrene. Secondly, asbestos fibers are more effective in benzo[a]pyrene transport than silicate.

Nickel-processing workers have increased risk for developing cancer in lung and nasal cavities [46]. It has been assumed that it was a result of the carcinogenicity of nickel; however, the distribution of lung cancer has not always followed a clear pattern of exposure to nickel compounds, but has been more related to dust exposure. Different observations in mining areas and smelters around the world have also been difficult to explain. A recent study of Langer et al. [23] indicates that nickel ore deposits around the world are frequently contaminated with asbestos. Lung cancer among these workers may be due, in part, to asbestos exposure. Animal models could be used to study the interactive effects between nickel and asbestos.

In Vitro Studies Using Cultured Tissues and Cells

The study of interaction between asbestos and cultured mammalian cells will lead to a better understanding of the pathogenic mechanisms of asbestos. Cytotoxicity and

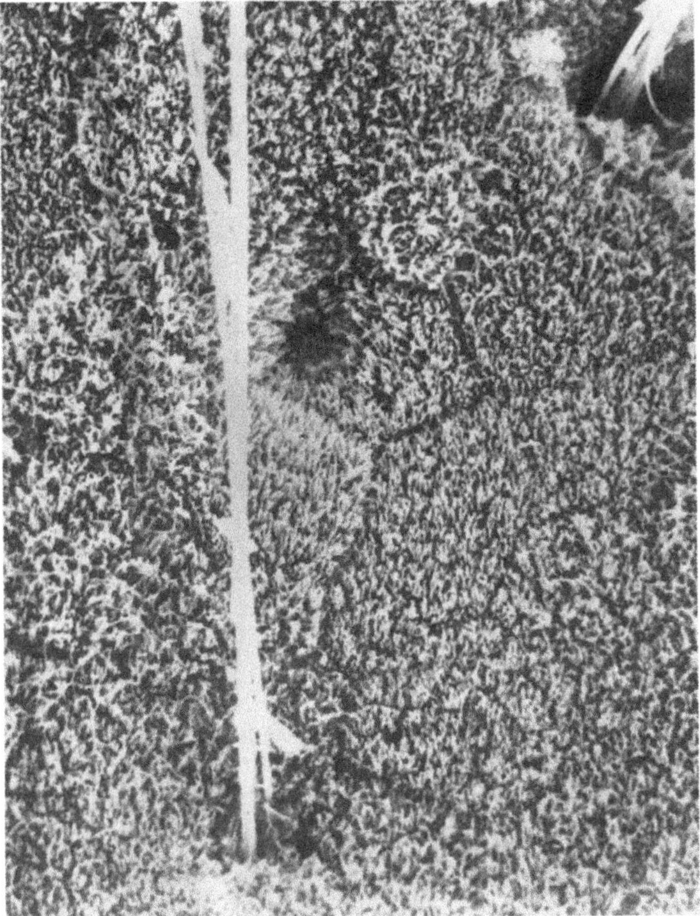

Fig. 1. Detail of tracheal surface 6 h after amosite fibers were added to the explants showing fibers protruding from the human bronchial epithelium. Magnification × 3,300

fibrinogenesis have been extensively studied in cultured cells. At the cellular level asbestos causes lysis of erythrocytes and is cytotoxic for macrophages, fibroblasts, and epithelioid cell lines [13, 33, 38]. The hemolytic potency and the effect of macrophages parallels fibrogenic activities of silica and asbestos in vivo. Silica and chrysotile are both toxic, while crocidolite and amosite have a relatively weak effect; however, their hemolytic activity can be enhanced by complement [30]. This difference has been related to magnesium content in their fiber [12]. The exact mechanism(s) of cell killing by asbestos is not clear. It has been suggested that cytotoxicity results from surface damage by asbestos of phagosomal membranes, and the damaged phagosomes then release lytic enzymes into the cytoplasm. There is, however, no quantitative correlation between these biological effects and the carcinogenic activity of asbestos. The most cytotoxic types of asbestos are not necessarily the most carcinogenic. However, Chamberlain and Brown [4] have reported that cytotoxic effects of mineral dusts on Chinese hamster V-79 and human lung A549 cells differ markedly from those

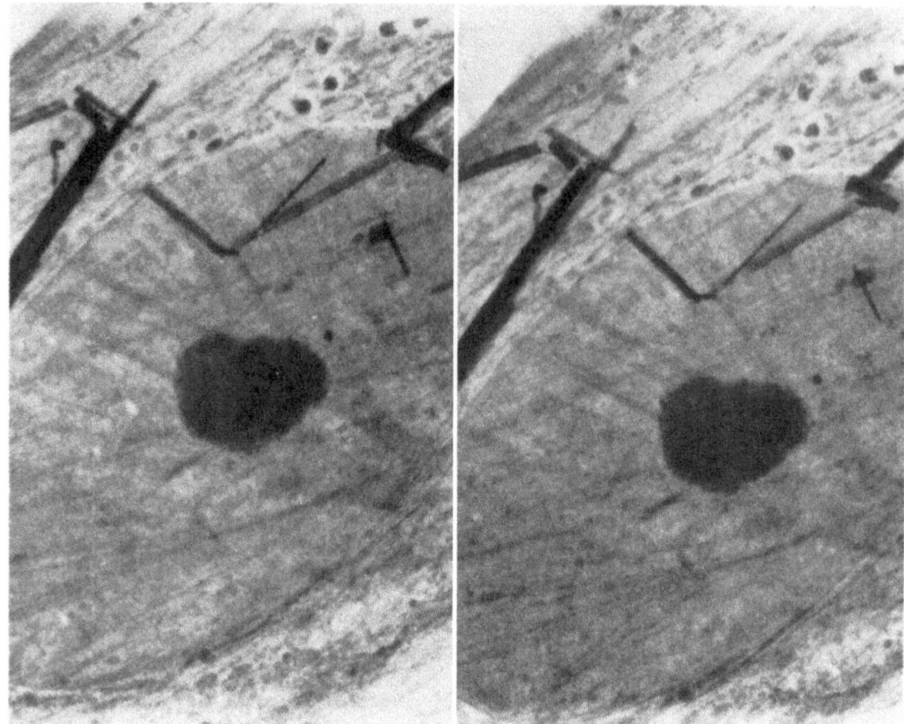

Fig. 2. A whole-cell preparation of human bronchial epithelium cell stained with 2% uranyl acetate and examined by high voltage electron microscopy. When the electron micrographs are viewed stereoscopically it is evident that some of the amosite fibers are located in the cytoplasm. Magnification × 4,000

in macrophage cultures; i.e., silica has little effect and the UICC asbestos dusts are very cytotoxic. They found a qualitative correlation between the cytotoxic effect of the dusts and the ability to induce mesothelioma after intrapleural injection of the dusts into rats. They suggest that the fibrous morphology of the dust is an important determinant of cytotoxicity.

Few reports concerning asbestos-induced chromosomal aberration and mutagenicity are available. Chromosomal breaks, gaps, deletions, and exchanges have been reported in Chinese hamster lung cells [19], Syrian hamster embryo cells [43], and Chinese hamster ovary cells [24] that have been exposed to asbestos fibers in vitro. Chromosomal changes were not induced by glass fibers of undetermined size. Huang [18] reported recently that phagocytized crocidolite fibers are weakly mutagenic at the hypoxanthine-guanine phosphoribosyl transferase locus in Chinese hamster lung cells.

Cultured explants permit studies on the biochemical and histopathological effects at the tissue level of biological organization. Since bronchial and tracheal explants retain both tissue-type specific structure and function in long-term culture [14], these cultured respiratory tract tissues are ideally suited for investigation of specific and general epithelial changes produced by asbestos. Exposure of cultured hamster trachea explants to crocidolite asbestos caused cytotoxic alterations, necrosis, and

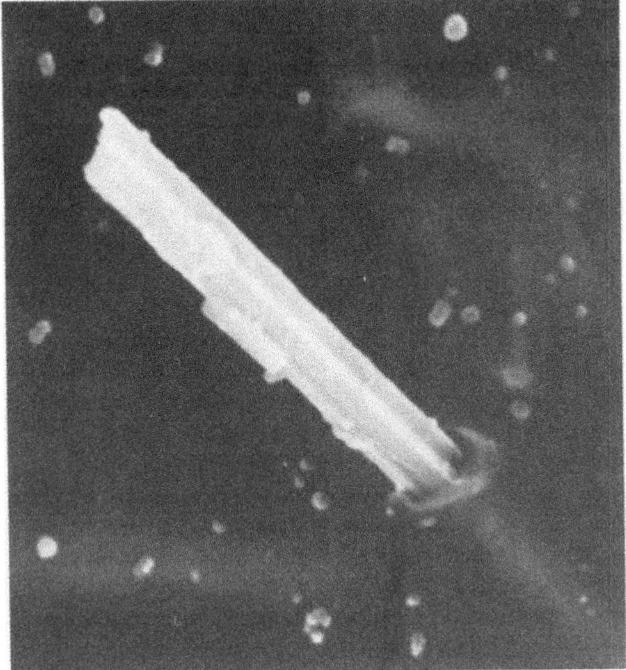

Fig. 3. Scanning electron micrograph demonstrating an amosite fiber that has partially entered an epithelial cell. Magnification × 15,000

desquamation of the epithelial cells, followed by hyperplasia and squamous metaplasia [31]. Crocidolite fibers were phagocytized by cells of the hyperplastic basal layer. The authors were also able to demonstrate that the fibers penetrated the mucosa into the submucosa in cultured trachea.

We have recently initiated investigations to examine the effects of asbestos fibers on cultured human trachea and bronchus, and cultured human epithelial cells. This culture system has been described previously [14, 25, 45]. An exclusive report from these experiments will be published later. Briefly, human bronchial tissues were obtained from either surgery or immediate autopsy. The tissues were kept at 4° C in L-15 culture medium for transport to the laboratory. Using sterile techniques, the tissues were dissected into explants of approximately 0.5 cm^2, placed in tissue culture dishes and incubated at 36.5° C on a rocker platform. Tissue explants were exposed to amosite asbestos by pipetting suspensions of asbestos fibers onto the epithelial surface. The explants were then submerged in medium in a stationary position for 2 h before continuous rocking on a moving platform. The culture medium was replaced with fresh medium without fibers the next day and then at 2-day intervals. In parallel studies, asbestos was added to cultures of epithelial cells. The next day, the medium was changed to medium without asbestos. Preliminary studies indicate that amosite asbestos causes focal lesions of hyperplasia and squamous metaplasia in cultured human bronchi and trachea. Asbestos fibers are found protruding from the bronchial epithelium shortly after exposure to asbestos (Fig. 1). Large fibers are usually removed by ciliary action, but occasionally fibers are observed on the ciliated epithelium 8 weeks or more after asbestos was added to the explants. Morphological studies show that fibers penetrate human bronchial epithelial cells. By analysis of

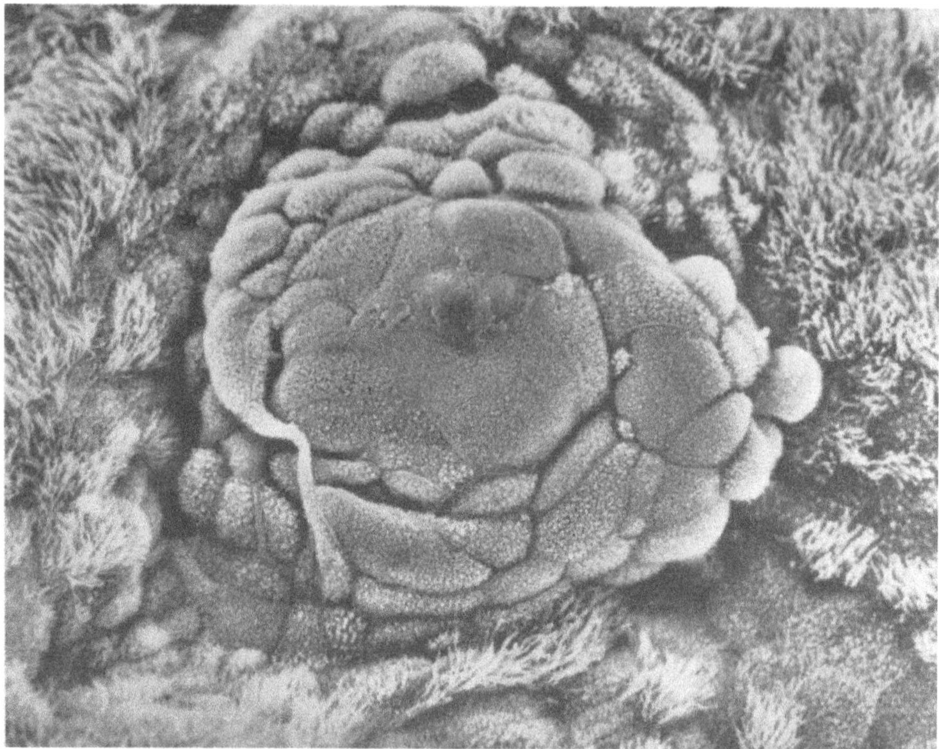

Fig. 4. Topographic view of a lesion from an explant 6 weeks after amosite (1,000 µg/ml) was precipitated on the explant. Normal ciliated tracheal epithelium is replaced by focal elevation of nonciliated cells with convex surfaces and numerous short microvilli. Magnification × 1,200

whole-cell preparations of bronchial epithelial cells by high-voltage electron microscopy and scanning electron microscopy, it was seen that short fibers (less than 12 µm) quickly penetrated the cells, whereas with longer fibers part of the asbestos fiber may remain outside the cell. Asbestos was present within the cells by 6 h (Fig. 2). It is well known that alveolar macrophages quickly phagocytize asbestos fibers and coat them with hemosiderin [47]. Exposed macrophages demonstrate increased surface activity and developed elongated fingerlike phagocytic processes on the surface surrounding the fiber [29]. In contrast, epithelial cells exposed to amosite showed no increased surface activity and the fibers were generally phagocytized end first with only a sleeve of membrane around them (Fig. 3). By scanning electron microscopy, epithelial lesions appear as focal elevation of nonciliated cells with microvilli and convex surfaces (Fig. 4). The development of lesions can be observed as early as 2 weeks after exposure to asbestos. In some places the normal cellular differentiation persisted. Atypia of these bronchial epithelial cells was manifested by cellular polymorphism, considerable variation in nuclear size, and nucleolar abnormalities (Fig. 5). Hyperplastic or metaplastic lesions were infrequently observed in the controls (Fig. 6). Studies are in progress to quantitate the frequency and tumorigenic potential of the epithelial lesions caused by different types of asbestos.

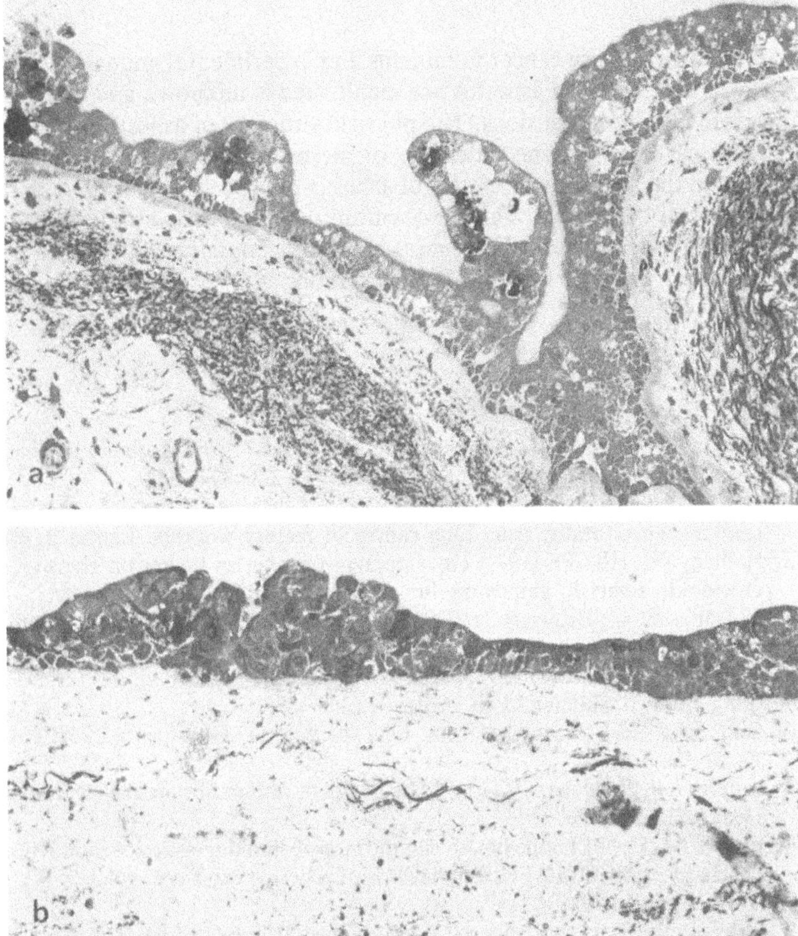

Fig. 5a, b. Absence of normal mucociliary differentiation 2 weeks after a single exposure to amosite fibers (100 µg/ml). Focal elevation of atypical non-ciliated cells, large polygonal cells, and loss of cellular polarity. Magnification × 130

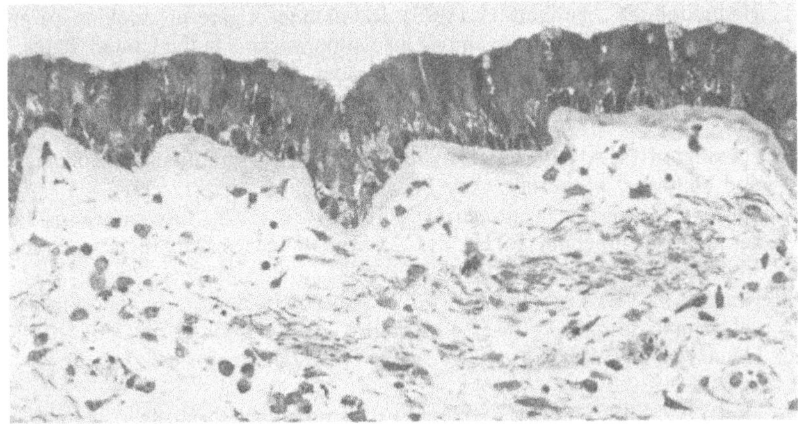

Fig. 6. Normal-appearing epithelium of control human bronchial explant 2 weeks after sham exposure. Magnification × 220

Conclusion

Asbestos fibers cause cancer in humans and experimental animals. The mechanism(s) by which the effects of asbestos are manifested is unknown and many of the findings suggest diverging conclusions. The physical structure of asbestos fiber is considered to be a critical factor in the induction of mesothelioma, while chemical factors may, because of the adsorptive capacity of asbestos, play a significant role in the etiology of bronchogenic carcinoma. The use of cultured human tissues and cells offers a valuable system for studying the mechanism(s) of carcinogenesis caused by asbestos at the tissue and cellular levels of biological organization.

References

1. Bayliss DL, Dement JM, Wagoner JK, Blejer HP (1976) Mortality pattern among fibrous glass production workers. Ann NY Acad Sci 271: 324−335
2. Berry G, Newhouse ML, Tubok M (1972) Combined effects of asbestos exposure and smoking on mortality from lung cancer in factory workers. Lancet 2: 476−478
3. Botham SK, Holt PF (1971) Development of asbestos bodies on amosite, chrysotile, and crocidolite fibers in guinea-pig lungs. J Pathol 105: 159−167
4. Chamberlain M, Brown RC (1978) The cytotoxic effects of asbestos and other mineral dust in tissue culture cell lines. Br J Exp Pathol 59: 183−189
5. Churg A, Warnock ML (1977) Analysis of the cores of ferruginous (asbestos) bodies from the general population. Lab Invest 37: 280−286
6. Doll R (1955) Mortality from lung cancer in asbestos workers. Br J Ind Med 12: 81−86
7. Enterline P, Henderson V (1975) The health of retired fibrous glass workers. Arch Environ Health 30: 113−116
8. Frank, AL (1979) Public health significance of smoking-asbestos interactions. In: Selikoff IJ, Hammond EC (eds) Health hazards of asbestos exposure, vol 330. NY Acad Sci, New York, pp 791−794
9. Gross P (1979) Is short-fibered asbestos dust a biological hazard? Arch Environ Health 29: 115−117
10. Gross P, de Treville RTP, Tolker EB, Kaschak M, Babyak MA (1967) Experimental asbestosis − the development of lung cancer in rats with pulmonary deposits of chrysotile asbestos dust. Arch Environ Health 15: 343−355
11. Hammond EC, Selikoff IJ (1973) Relation of cigarette smoking to risk of death of asbestos-associated disease among insulation workers in the United States. In: Bogovski P, Gilson JC, Timbrell V et al. (eds) Biological effects of asbestos. IARC, Lyon, p 312
12. Harrington JS, Miller K, Macnab G (1971) Hemolysis of asbestos. Environ Res 4: 95−117
13. Harrington JS, Allison AC, Badami PV (1975) Mineral fibers: chemical, physicochemical and biological properties. Adv Pharmacol Chemother 12: 291−402
14. Harris CC, Autrup H, Stoner GD, Trump BF (1978) Carcinogenesis studies in human respiratory epithelium. In: Harris CC (ed) Pathogenesis and therapy of lung cancer, vol 10. Marcel Dekker, New York, pp 559−607
15. Henderson VL, Enterline PE (1979) Asbestos exposure: factors associated with excess cancer and respiratory disease mortality. Ann NY Acad Sci 330: 117−126
16. Hendry NW (1965) The geology, occurrences, and major uses of asbestos. Ann NY Acad Sci 132: 12−22
17. Holt PF, Mills J, Young DK (1966) Experimental asbestosis in the guinea-pig. J Pathol Bacteriol 92: 185−195

18. Huang SL (1979) Amosite, chrysotile and crocidolite asbestos are mutagenic in Chinese hamster lung cells. Mutat Res 68: 265
19. Huang SL, Saggioro D, Michelmann H, Malling HV (1978) Genetic effects of crocidolite asbestos in Chinese hamster lung cells. Mutat Res 57: 225–232
20. International agency for research on cancer annual report (1978) Lyon
21. Kogan FM, Guselnikova NA, Gulevskaya MR (1972) Cancer mortality rate among workers in the asbestos industry of the Urals. Gig Sanit 37: 29–32
22. Lakowicz JR, Hylden JL (1978) Asbestos-mediated membrane uptake of benzo[a]pyrene observed by fluorescence spectroscopy. Nature 275: 446–448
23. Langer AM, Rohl AN, Selikoff IJ (1980) Asbestos as a cofactor in carcinogenesis among nickel-processing workers. Science 209: 420
24. LaVappa KS, Fu MM, Epstein SS (1975) Cytogenetic studies on chrysotile asbestos. Environ Res 10: 165–173
25. Lechner JF, Haugen A, Autrup H et al. (1981) Clonal growth of cultured epithelial cells from normal adult human bronchus. Cancer Res 41: 2294–2304
26. Lynch KM, Smith WA (1935) Pulmonary asbestosis. III. Carcinoma of lung in asbesto-silicosis. Am J Cancer 24: 56–64
27. Lynch KM, McIver FA, Cain JR (1957) Pulmonary tumors in mice exposed to asbestos dust. AMA Arch Ind Health 15: 207
28. Martischnig KM, Newell DJ, Barnsley WC, Cowan WK, Feinmann EL, Oliver E (1977) Unsuspected exposure to asbestos and bronchogenic carcinoma. Br Med J 1: 746–749
29. McLemore TL, Mace ML, Roggli V et al. (1980) Asbestos body phagocytosis by human free alveolar macrophages. Cancer Lett 9: 85
30. Miller K, Harington JS, Macnab G (1972) Effects of asbestos on macrophages in culture. S Afr Med J 46: 819
31. Mossmann BT, Kessler JB, Ley BW, Craighead JE (1977) Interaction of crocidolite asbestos with hamster respiratory mucosa in organ culture. Lab Invest 36: 131–139
32. National Toxicology Program (1980) First annual report on carcinogens, vol II. U.S. Public Health Service, Washington DC, p 51
33. Neugut AI, Eisenberg D, Silverstein M, Pulkrabek P, Weinstein IB (1978) Effects of asbestos on epithelioid cell lines. Environ Res 17: 256
34. Nordmann M, Sorge A (1941) Lungenkrebs durch Asbeststaub im Tierversuch. Z Krebsforsch 51: 168
35. Pyler LN, Shabad LM (1973) Some results of experimental studies in asbestos carcinogenesis. In: Bogovski P, Gilson JC, Timbrell V et al. (eds) Biological effects of asbestos. IARC, Lyon, p 99ff
36. Reeves AL, Puro HE, Smith RB, Vorwald AJ (1971) Experimental asbestos carcinogenesis. Environ Res 4: 496
37. Reeves AL, Puro HE, Smith RG (1974) Inhalation carcinogenesis from various forms of asbestos. Environ Res 8: 178–202
38. Richards RJ, Jacoby F (1976) Light microscope studies on the effects of chrysotile asbestos and fiber glass on the morphology and reticulin formation of cultured lung fibroblasts. Environ Res 11: 112–121
39. Selikoff IJ, Hammond EC (1979) Asbestos and smoking. JAMA 242: 458–459
40. Selikoff IJ, Hammond EC, Churg J (1968) Asbestos exposure, smoking, and neoplasia. JAMA 204: 106–112
41. Selikoff IJ, Hammond EC, Churg J (1972) Carcinogenicity of amosite asbestos. Arch Environ Health 25: 183–186
42. Selikoff IJ, Lee DHK (1978) Asbestos and disease. Academic Press, New York, p 307
43. Sincock A, Seabright M (1975) Induction of chromosome changes in Chinese hamster cells by exposure to asbestos fibers. Nature 257: 56–58
44. Stanton MF, Wrench C (1972) Mechanisms of mesothelioma induction with asbestos and fibrous glass. J Natl Cancer Inst 48: 797–821

45. Stoner GD, Katoh Y, Foidart JM, Myers GA, Harris CC (1980) Identification and culture of human bronchial epithelial cells. In: Harris CC, Trump BF, Stoner GD (eds) Methods in cell biology, vol 21A. Academic Press, New York, p 15
46. Sunderman PW (1979) Carcinogenicity and anticarcinogenicity of metal compounds. In: Emmelot P, Kriek E (eds) Environmental carcinogenesis. Elsevier/North-Holland Biomed Press, Amsterdam, p 165
47. Suzuki Y, Churg J (1969) Structure and development of the asbestos body. Am J Pathol 55:79–107
48. Topping DC, Nettesheim P (1980) Two-stage carcinogenesis studies with asbestos in Fisher 344 rats. J Natl Cancer Inst 65:627–630
49. Topping DC, Nettesheim P, Martin DH (to be published) Toxic and tumorigenic effects of asbestos in tracheal mucosa. Environ Pathol Toxicol
50. Wagner JC, Berry G, Timbrell V (1973) Mesotheliomata in rats after inoculation with asbestos and other materials. Br J Cancer 28:173–185
51. Wagner JC, Berry G, Skidmore JW, Timbrell V (1974) The effects of the inhalation of asbestos in rats. Br J Cancer 29:252–269
52. Warnock ML, Churg AM (1975) Association of asbestos and bronchogenic carcinoma in a population with low asbestos exposure. Cancer 35:1236–1242
53. Whitwell F, Newhouse ML, Bennett DR (1974) A study of the histological cell types of lung caner in workers suffering from asbestosis in the United Kingdom. Br J Ind Med 31:298–303

The Contribution of Uranium Miners to Lung Cancer Histogenesis

G. Saccomanno

St. Mary's Hospital, Grand Junction, CO, USA

Uranium mining on the Colorado Plateau started as an aggressive industry in 1950. At that time, little was known about the carcinogenic hazards of uranium mining except for the high incidence of cancer in the Old World uranium mining industry of Schneeberg in Germany and Joachimsthal in Czechoslovakia during the 19th century. Suspicions were voiced and predictions made that there could be a high incidence of lung cancer in our uranium mining population.

Duncan Holaday, then with the U.S. Public Health Service, encouraged government agencies to initiate studies on work level month (WLM) accumulation exposures, and personally researched extensively on modalities of measuring WLM [3, 4]. Furthermore, he realized and convincingly suggested that the most effective method of lowering WLM exposure was to improve mine ventilation. His persuasive manner won the support of the industry in initiating programs to correct the deficiency in a scientific way. Others, of course, contributed by way of engineering knowledge and instrumentation, but Mr. Holaday was the one who actively convinced industry, labor, and government to support mine ventilation. He was successful in the introduction and advancement of the science of radon daughter understanding and control. He also encouraged government agencies (U.S. Public Health) to initiate epidemiological studies. However, no one was aware at the time of the many situations which, retrospectively, would be problems in evaluating health liabilities. Populations could be studied epidemiologically, but no one realized that the radon daughter exposure would decrease rapidly with improved ventilation. Moreover, the amount of radon daughter exposure to miners prior to the initiation of studies would, at best, be difficult to estimate because of inadequate instrumentation and lack of mine readings. A large error, probably on the low side, was a good guess. Little was known of the problem and even less was done in evaluating the effects of radiation on those exposed, but still Duncan Holaday had the foresight to initiate a program of epidemiology under the direction of Dr. Victor Archer.

In 1955, Dr. Victor Archer began his study under the support of the U.S. Public Health Service to identify a group of 3,414 white and 761 nonwhite uranium miners. The project consisted of performing annual physical examinations, collecting sputum samples on an annual basis, and initiating a program of radon measurements in uranium mines. Meanwhile, our own interest had been stimulated by physicians of Mesa County and occasional uranium miners who came to St. Mary's Hospital for diagnosis and treatment of lung neoplasia. When Dr. Archer inquired about our willingness to participate in conducting sputum cytology and tumor collection on the uranium miners, we were very much interested and agreed to take part in this program.

A joint effort was then developed with financial support by the U.S. Public Health Service. Dr. O. Auerbach agreed to undertake the horrendous task of making serial block sections of all the lung cases who might develop cancer, and to join us and others in reading the histology of these tumors. The first contract to perform autopsies on uranium miners and initiate the formation of the uranium miner lung cancer library, which now houses 312 lung cancer cases and approximately 200,000 sputum study findings, was signed in 1957.

In 1950–1955 it all seemed very simple: cancer of the lung could be diagnosed early by chest X-ray, and/or sputum cytology, done annually or semiannually. It was though that if these studies could be implemented on a significant number of active miners, the disease might be kept under control. It was anticipated that the lesions could be identified by either or both modalities and that the majority of the cases could be treated and cured for the benefit of the miners. Actually the avenues which our studies followed were to lead us away from this objective. The facts available then should have alerted us to the many circumstances that proved this path unyielding. First, as we reported in 1964, the majority of the tumors (77%) were of the small cell type, and even today this disease is inoperable. Second, sputum cytology yielded such a poor quality slide that it defied a correct diagnosis and proved to be no more than a nominal procedure.

An interesting series of events led us to develop the art of sputum cytology. Most of our experimentation in this endeavor arose from the fact that it would be almost impossible to make direct sputum smear slides from miners who, at the end of a working shift and anxious to get home, would be challenged to give a sputum sample. They were reluctant to take an additional half hour for aerosolization, and we felt that after aerosolization under these rushed conditions, the material would be inadequate to make an accurate diagnosis.

Development of Sputum Cytology Technology

The first question to be considered in developing this technology was: can a fluid fixative be found which would preserve the specimen sufficiently well to collect samples at the mines and return the fixed samples to the laboratory for processing? This, today, seems like an absurd question, but at the time, no fixative had been found to fix cellular elements in sputum properly. Moreover, the problem really related directly to the mucus in the sputum. Alcohol in strengths thought to be strong enough to kill bacteria resulted in coagulation of the mucoprotein. Sectioning the coagulum resulted in poor cytological preparations. The hunt and peck technology left much to be desired on single cases and proved totally inadequate for a large number of samples. A solution had to be found.

First, a series of ethyl alcohol dilutions were tested with strengths of 20%, 30%, 40%, 50%, 60%, 70%, and 80%. The 60% ethyl alcohol did not coagulate the mucoproteins, but seemed to be less preferable than the 50% alcohol which did not shrink the cells and still resulted in a clear sputum smear. Lesser strengths of 40% and 30% also seemed to stay the growth of bacteria, but were considered inadequate because addition of the sputum specimen added 15–20 ml of fluid volume, further diluting the alcohol strength. Carbowax 1540 U.K. was added as a beneficial fixing agent. It has been suspected of coating the cells, preventing shrinkage, and also allows drying of the slides prior to staining.

The second concern was the mucus fibers of the sputum sample. As mentioned above, the mucus fibers consist of mucoproteins which begin to coagulate at strengths of 70% ethyl alcohol and completely coagulate when added to 100% ethyl alcohol. The thought of blending the specimen with a Waring blender was a good one. Blending sputum samples at 21,000 rpm does not damage the cells if it is limited to 5−10 s. This usually liquifies the mucus by mixing in the alcohol. Teasing a sputum sample with a sharp instrument reveals varying thickness of the mucus fibers. Some are very thick and others are very fine. Blending the sputum samples seems to liquify the majority of the mucus fibers, leaving only the thick fibers, which are cut into short segments by the blending blades. Some of the cut fibers can be found in the smears from patients with chronic obstructive pulmonary disease, who usually show the most tenacious thick mucus fibers. Centrifugation of the specimen allows the cells in the sputum suspension to be separated from the fibers in solution. This technology was published in 1963 [6]. Some refinements have been added, but the technique remains basically as published and is now widely used in many hospitals.

Radon Daughter Exposure Evaluation

Our program of uranium miner studies was rather well established by 1960. Our objectives, at that time, were few: to collect lungs from uranium miners who died, regardless of the cause of death, to collect bone tissues for lead and polonium studies [1, 2], and finally to collect sputum samples once a year from as many miners as possible who wished to participate. This was done primarily to identify patients with early neoplasia, but we also hoped to learn more and more about lung cancer, cell types, how tumors developed over time, etc.

No one anticipated the many variables which would evolve in epidemiological data analysis of the effects of radon daughters on the uranium miner. Some of the variables influencing the data analysis of this work exposure were as follows:

1) The radon daughter levels in the mines varied not only over time (progressively decreasing from levels in some mines of over 50 WL to less than 0.3 WL), but also from mine to mine or even from stope to stope. The larger mines reduced the WL as rapidly as was economically feasible, but the smaller mines were faced with economic problems, ventilating cost exceeding at times the value of extracting a small ore body. Large quantities of cold air during the winter created a cold working place and caused shutdown of ventilating fans, which varied the WL.

2) The age of the workers and duration of the individual miner exposure had to be considered. A uranium miner initiating his employment at age 50 certainly would not receive the same injury or effect from radon exposure as one starting at age 16.

3) Whether a uranium miner smoked cigarettes in and out of the mine, and if so, whether he was a light or heavy smoker, had to be taken into account.

4) The accuracy of the records kept of the exposure levels was a relevant aspect.

5) The size of the population exposed had its implications. Investigation of a large population group usually results in meaningful data analysis, but does not take into

consideration the individual exposed whose sensitivity and life are at stake. Therefore, lumping data is equitable to neither the miner nor the mining industry.

These are only a few of the problems making effective analysis of the uranium mining exposure to radiation very difficult.

We have little information on the total population exposed to radon daughters in uranium mining. A conservative guess is that the total uranium mining population over the last 40 years is in the region of 100,000 miners, but it might be significantly more than this. One must also ask: should one who mined uranium for 10 days during 1950–1960 be considered among the exposed population, particularly if during this period he was exposed to 50 WL per day? This is a relatively large daily dose. Should he be evaluated as receiving the same radiation as one working for 1,000 days in the latter part of the 1970s at 0.5 WL? Supposing the former or the latter smoked or did not — if one developed neoplasia, how would these variables affect the interpretation? Our laws allow that the mining company in which the uranium miner was last employed is liable for compensation to the miner. One mining company employed a miner provisionally, pending sputum studies. After 4 days of employment, the sputum report indicated that the miner had a cancer of the lung. The court ruled the company liable for this man's tumor. The judgment was for $22,000.00. This patient probably had had the tumor for several years before he was employed. Was this a fair judgment? Finally, even if the total number of uranium miners exposed were known, we still would not know with any degree of accuracy how many uranium miners developed neoplasia. Our library contains 312 cases of lung cancer among uranium miners, but this may represent 25%, 50%, or 75% of all the uranium miners who developed lung cancer.

Cancer of the Lung: Incidence and Cell Type

It has not been determined conclusively that radon daughter exposure causes any other cell type of lung tumor than the so-called small cell (oat cell) carcinoma. Some writers have presented data suggesting that the epidermoid carcinomas and adenocarcinomas are also increased if the uranium miner is a cigarette smoker. This is probably correct in miners who had exposures above 300 WLM and were cigarette smokers. It is not proven conclusively in lesser exposures and since the incidence is increased in cigarette smokers, the cigarette smoking is probably the principal primary cause of these kinds of carcinoma. At the same time there is rather conclusive additional evidence that oat cell carcinomas are increasing among nonminers who are heavy cigarette smokers (3–4 packs or more per day); this seems particularly so among women. Nonetheless, radon daughter exposure in heavy doses unquestionably has caused oat cell carcinoma in the uranium miner.

The incidence of oat cell cancer of the lung has decreased over the last 20 years and presently accounts for slightly more than 22% of the uranium miners developing neoplasia, compared to 17% in the nonmining cigarette smoking population (Fig. 1). Cigarette smoking remains a most potent carcinogenic agent in the uranium miner (Table 1).

We have had only 14 cases of lung cancer among nonsmoking uranium miners, and of these, eight (57%) were of the oat cell type (Tables 1 and 2).

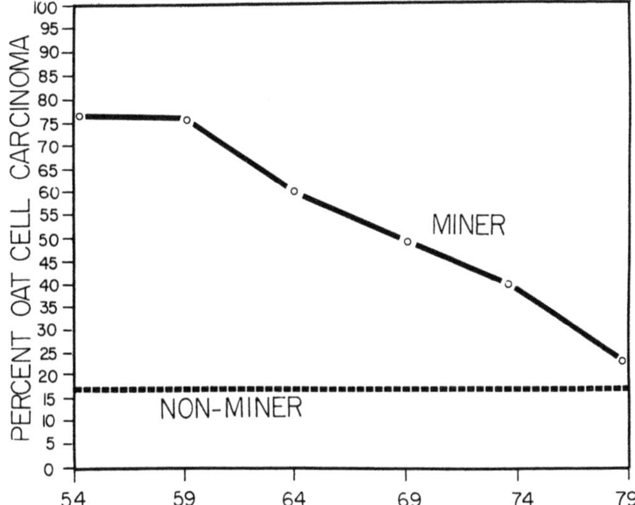

Fig. 1. Percentage of oat cell carcinoma among 292 cases of lung cancer in uranium miners. Colorado Plateau 1954–1979

Table 1. Three hundred and twelve (312) cancers of the lung in uranium miners related to smoking and nonsmoking; ratio of 60% smokers, 40% nonsmokers; Colorado Plateau 1954–1980

Smoking status	Expected	Observed
Smoker	187	277
Nonsmoker	125	14
Unknown		21

Table 2. Three hundred and twelve (312) cancers of the lung in uranium miners related to smoking and nonsmoking, age at death, and tumor type; Colorado Plateau 1954–1980

Smoking status		Average age at death (years)
Smokers:		
Oat cell	128	54
Non-oat cell	149	58
Total	277	56.5
Nonsmokers:		
Oat cell	8	48
Non-oat cell	6	53.5
Total	14	50.5
Unknown:		
Oat cell	5	56.5
Non-oat cell	16	59
Total	21	58

It is also interesting to note that the nonsmoking uranium miners who developed tumors died at an average age of 50 years 6 months. The cigarette smokers who also mined and developed oat cell carcinoma died at an average age of 54 years. The average age at death for nonsmokers who died of oat cell tumors was 48 years, while for those with epidermoid and other tumors it was 58 years in the case of smokers and 53 years 6 months in the case of nonsmokers. This implies that patients highly susceptible to the development of lung neoplasia may be so regardless of their smoking habits or that tumor induction probably occurs before the cigarette contributory factor comes into play. Some writers have suggested that cigarette smoking enhances tumor development, and that nonsmokers develop tumor at an older age. Our data on the miners do not support this thesis. One more concern is that while an oat cell tumor develops very rapidly, the other types of primary lung tumor take longer. Squamous cell tumors, in particular, take several years to develop.

Lung Cancer Histogenesis:
Sequential Squamous Cell Metaplasia, Benign and Premalignant

The phenomenon of squamous cell metaplasia progresses over time and ultimately develops into neoplasia of the lung in about 15−20 years [7]. This is certainly true in the development of squamous cell carcinoma, and some evidence suggests that large cell undifferentiated carcinoma, adenocarcinoma, and adenosquamous cell carcinoma also develop in this manner. This feature of metaplasia is also noted in scar tumors giving rise to squamous cell carcinoma, bronchoalveolar carcinoma, and adenocarcinoma elements surrounding a central scar. However, the majority of the squamous cell metaplasias are seen in nonneoplastic reactions of the lung.

Although one focus of squamous cell metaplasia may develop into neoplasia, which can be identified cytologically and histologically, patients with neoplasia also shed a variety of metaplastic squamous cells. This is demonstrated in the cytogram of a lung cancer patient which shows neoplastic cells as well as an abundance of mild, moderate, and marked (severe) atypical squamous cell metaplasia (Fig. 2). One may conclude that these cells have the potential for neoplasia given sufficient time to develop into tumor.

Figure 3 represents 38 cases of uranium miners identified initially as having benign cytology with varying degrees of atypia, and who were followed over time. All eventually developed histologically proven neoplasia. Comparison of these cases reveals several variables in the development of neoplasia. The ages ranged from 38 to 75 years, but the majority of the cases developed these tumors in their fifth or sixth decade. The time which each case spent in each phase of atypia and the duration of the carcinoma in situ also varied considerably. Some of the cases showing squamous cell carcinoma also developed oat cell cancer which cut short the period of maturity of the squamous cell lesion. Figure 4 shows the average of 33 cases with the age range in each phase of the developing tumor.

Squamous cell metaplasia, however, is found in the young and the old and does not always represent a benign to malignant process, but more frequently a nonspecific bronchial epithelial reaction which is readily reversible with disappearance of the toxic, infectious, or inflammatory factor which caused it. For example, Figs. 5 and 6 reveal that in uranium miners as well as in nonminers, the proportion of squamous cell metaplasia is higher among cigarette smokers than nonsmokers. Further, about 12%

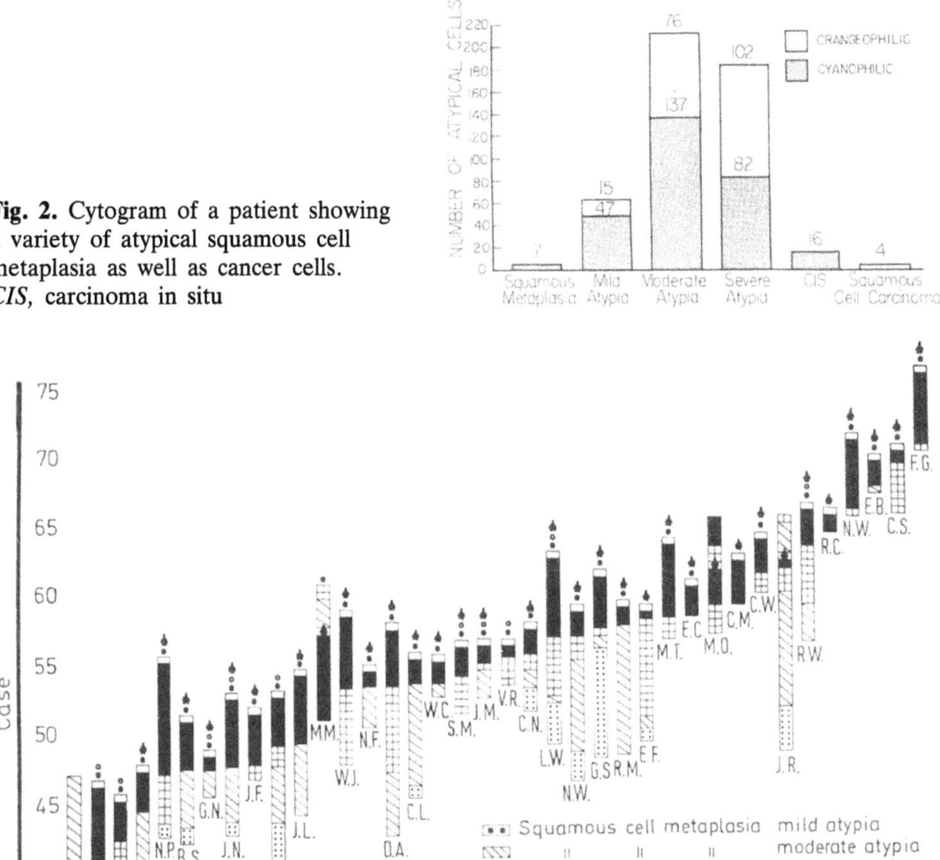

Fig. 2. Cytogram of a patient showing a variety of atypical squamous cell metaplasia as well as cancer cells. *CIS,* carcinoma in situ

Fig. 3. Development of carcinoma of the lung (epidermoid type)

of the cases showing moderate atypia progress to marked atypia each year and eventually to neoplasia. Therefore the majority of cases of moderate atypia either remain moderate, or revert to a lower degree of atypia, or completely disappear. This must be a relatively mobile phenomenon in the lung, and the reasons for this are very poorly understood.

The phenomenon of atypical squamous cell metaplasia, which progresses to neoplasia over time, introduces many systemic as well as local reactions. Nasiell [5], in a retrospective study on these cellular changes using the Feulgen DNA assessment stain, presented evidence of nuclear DNA chromosomal changes of polypoidy, even in the early stages of development (moderate atypia) to some degree, and becoming more abnormal in marked atypia and carcinoma in situ. This seems to be a local cellular reaction, but may be related to systemic abnormalities as demonstrated immunologically.

                                                                G. Saccomanno

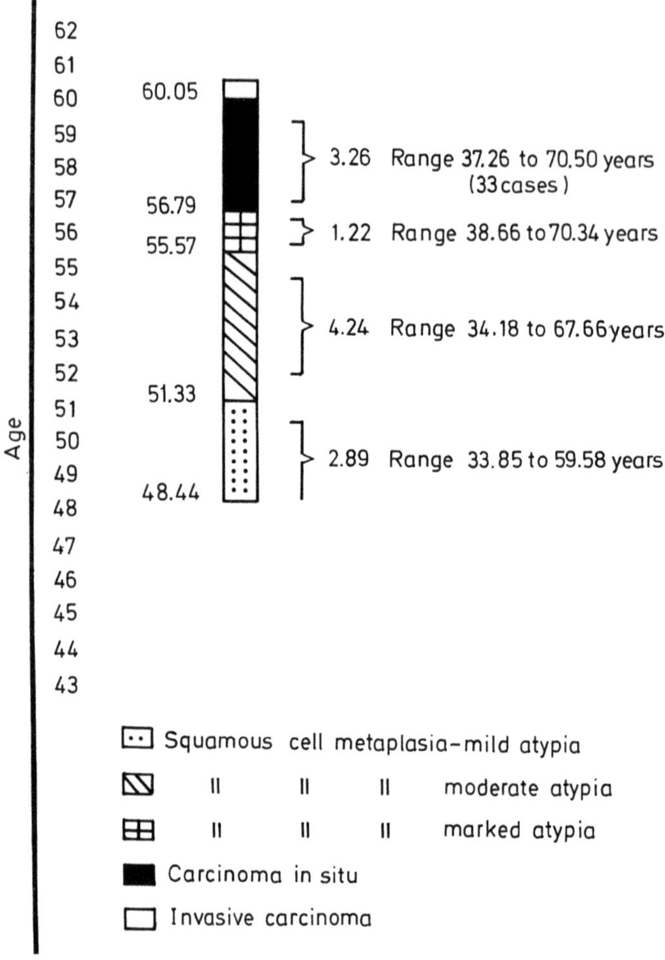

Fig. 4. Development of carcinoma of the lung. Average case (epidermoid carcinoma)

Gross (personal communication), using the T cell analysis, rosette inhibition test, and phytohemagglutinin test in patients with squamous cell metaplasia, showed that some degree of immunological impairment was evident in moderate atypia, but more pronounced in marked atypia, carcinoma in situ, and invasive carcinoma. The cellular change noted in the progression of atypia to neoplasia is probably a complex mechanism visible cytologically in shed metaplastic cells from the lung, and is possibly the product of an altered systemic immunological surveillance process. This certainly necessitates more in-depth research, not only into the chemistry of these abnormal cell changes, but also into how this relates to the body's immune system.

Further, studies on the significance of squamous cell metaplasia are presently in progress. A retrospective computerized study is under way which will assess the significance of moderate atypical squamous cell metaplasia when found in uranium miners. The computer analysis will relate this degree of atypia to numerous factors such as age, mining experience (WLM accumulation), smoking history, and other

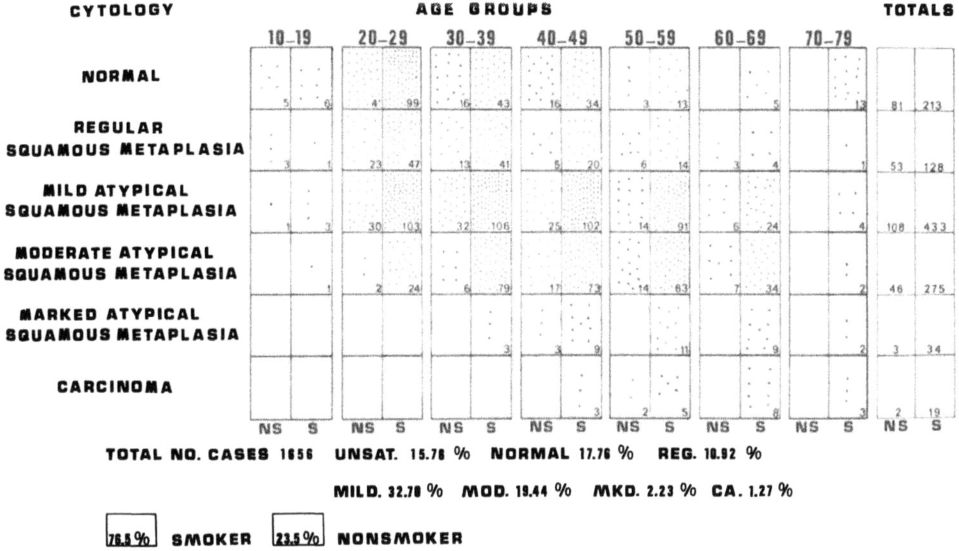

Fig. 5. Pulmonary cytology among uranium miners

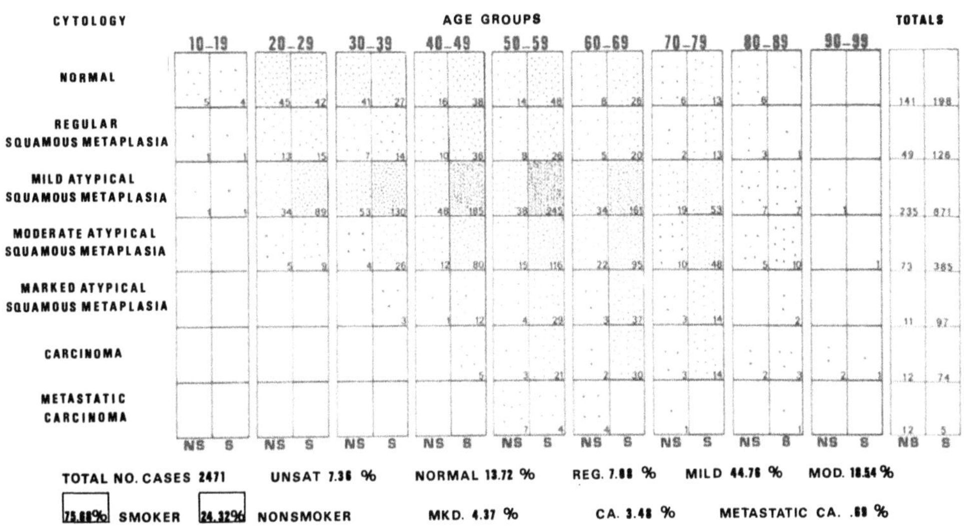

Fig. 6. Pulmonary cytology among nonminers

factors. We hope this analysis will lead to a better understanding of how and why tumors develop, and of the significance of this degree of atypia when it does not progress to neoplasia. Possibly some light will be shed on how this process, both benign and malignant, relates to the immune system.

Much knowledge regarding the development of lung cancer has depended on the contribution of the uranium miner who has been willing to cooperate in the collection of data upon himself, in the hope that, someday, lung cancer can be cured.

References

1. Archer VE, Black SC, Saccomanno G (1967) Urine and tissue content of ^{210}Pb and [210]Po in uranium miners. Diagnosis and treatment of deposited radionuclides. In: Proceedings of a symposium in Richland, Washington, 15−17 May 1967
2. Black SC, Archer VE, Dixon WC, Saccomanno G (1968) Correlation of radiation exposure and lead 210 in uranium miners. Health Phys 14:81−93
3. Holaday DA (1959) Radiation exposure in uranium mines and mills. Hearings on employee radiation hazards and workmen's compensation before the Subcommittee on Research and Development of the Joint Committee on Atomic Energy, Eighty-sixth Congress, March 10−19, 1959. US Government Printing Office, Washington, DC
4. Holaday DA, Rushing DE, Coleman RD, Woolrich PF, Kusnetz HL, Bale WF (1957) Control of radon and daughters in uranium mines and calculations on biologic effects. Public Health Service Publication 494. US Government Printing Office, Washington, DC
5. Nasiell M (1978) Cytomorphological grading and Feulgen DNA − analysis of metaplastic and neoplastic bronchial cells. Cancer 41:1511−1521
6. Saccomanno G, Saunders RP, Ellis H, Archer VE, Wood BG, Beckler PA (1963) Concentration of carcinoma or atypical cells in sputum. Acta Cytol 7:305−310
7. Saccomanno G, Archer VE, Auerbach O, Saunders RP, Brennan LM (1974) Development of carcinoma of the lung as reflected in exfoliated cells. Cancer 33:256−270

_Pathogenesis of Bronchial Carcinoma,
with Special Reference to Morphogenesis
and the Influence on the Bronchial Mucosa
of 20-Methylcholanthrene and Cigarette Smoking_

M. Nasiell, E. Carlens, G. Auer, Y. Hayata, H. Kato,
C. Konaka, V. Roger, K. Nasiell, and I. Enstad

Sabbatsberg Hospital, Departments of Pathology and Cytology, Box 6401,
S-11382 Stockholm, Sweden

It is generally assumed that squamous cell carcinoma is preceded by a series of progressive epithelial changes. The importance of pathogenetic studies is based on the fact that diagnosis and treatment of preinvasive or early invasive lesions can stop the development of epithelial tumors.

Epithelial Injury – Metaplasia – Atypia

A model for the pathogenesis of bronchogenic carcinoma with similarities to that of cervical carcinoma has been set up [27, 28]. This model includes epithelial injury, squamous metaplasia, various degrees of atypical metaplasia (dysplasia), carcinoma in situ, and invasive carcinoma (Fig. 1). The initiation phase seems to be characterized by an epithelial injury with basal cell hyperplasia [17] or cleavage – slit formation of the bronchial epithelium (Figs. 2, 3), with heavy loss (exfoliation) of degenerated columnar cells resulting in an unprotected, nonciliated, low epithelium (Fig. 4) [22, 24, 25]. Several studies and reports of these sequential changes have given further support to the suggested pathogenetic model [3, 8, 9, 35, 45, 46, 49]. An abundance of degenerated columnar cells are found in the corresponding sputum preparations. This cytological phenomenon was denominated abnormal columnar cell findings (ACCF) [24] (Fig. 5). The concept includes also Papanicolaou's ciliocytophthoria phenomenon (CCP) [34]. The resulting low nonciliated epithelium with its unprotected surface must

Early epithelial injury
↓
Squamous metaplasia (reversible
↓
Atypical metaplasia/dysplasia (probably reversible)
(mild ⟶ moderate ⟶ severe)
↓
Carcinoma in situ (reversible?)
↓
Early invasive carcinoma (irreversible)
↓
Invasive carcinoma

Fig. 1. Pathogenesis of bronchogenic carcinoma

Recent Results in Cancer Research, Vol. 82
© Springer-Verlag Berlin · Heidelberg 1982

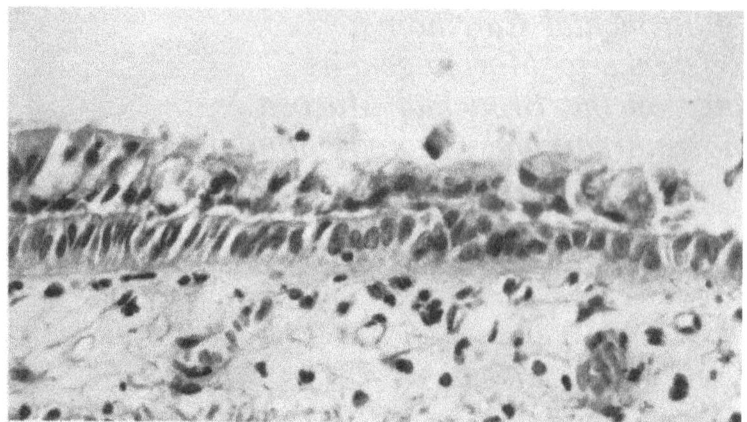

Fig. 2. Slit formation in the bronchial epithelium. The columnar surface cells show degenerative changes − a "low" epithelium is formed under the slit. Van Gieson × 250

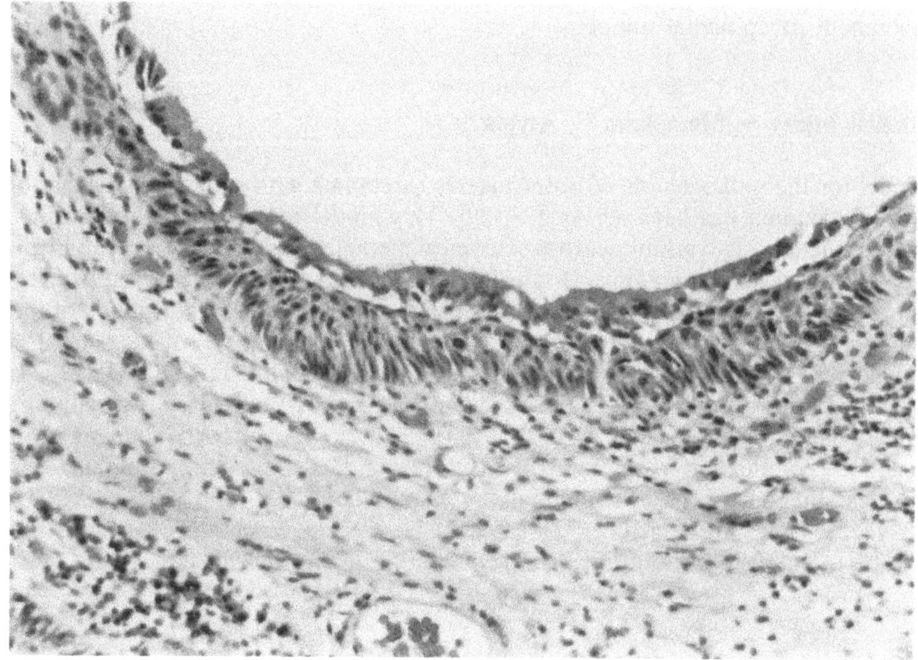

Fig. 3. Slit formation. The surface cells are degenerated and the underlying epithelium shows transitional squamous metaplastic changes. Hematoxylin-eosin × 155. Courtesy of Dr. L. B. Woolner, Rochester, USA

be sensitive to carcinogens in the mucus, which will not be removed properly. These observations have been confirmed by Hilding's and Stenbäck's experimental studies [8, 9, 45, 46]. The low epithelium then develops into a transitional or squamous metaplastic epithelium (Figs. 6−8) [22]. Table 1 shows that squamous metaplasia was found in 45% of the cases in a series of 211 patients with ACCF, and bronchial

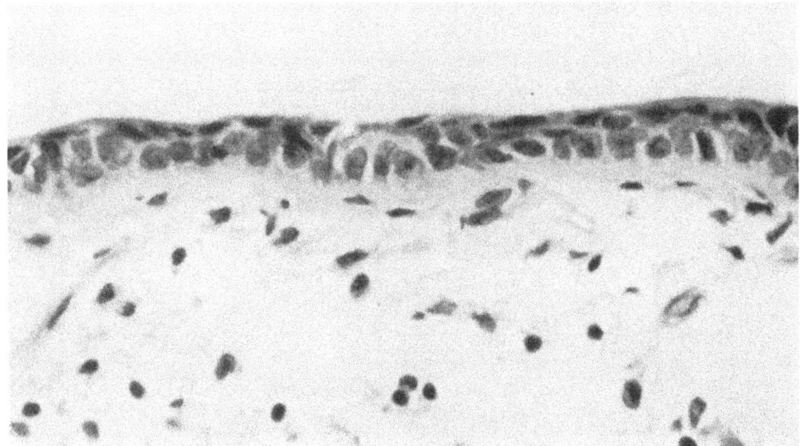

Fig. 4. Low nonciliated epithelium. There are no ciliated cells. Several surface cells are elongated. Van Gieson × 250

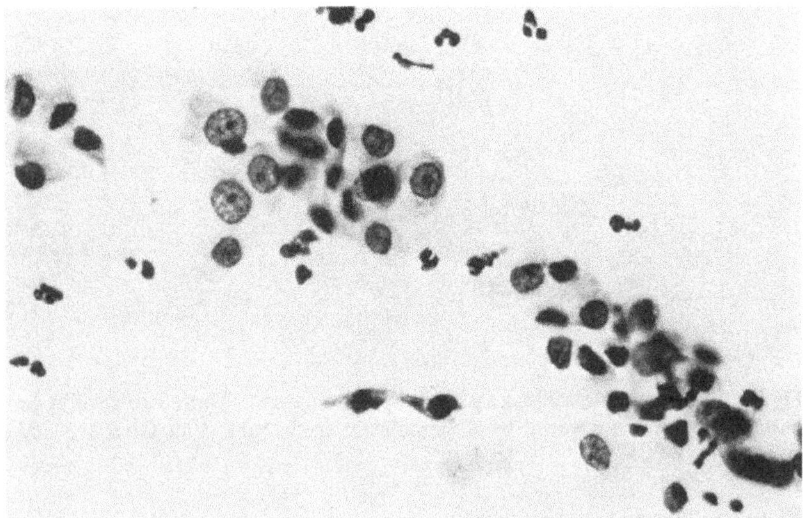

Fig. 5. Numerous degenerated columnar cells in a sputum sample (ACCF). Papanicolaou stain × 248

carcinoma in 39%. Only 16% of the 211 patients with ACCF had neither squamous metaplasia nor carcinoma. These results may indicate a close relationship between the epithelial injury, i.e., slit formation, ACCF, and squamous metaplasia as well as bronchial cancer [22, 24]. Figure 7 also illustrates a phenomenon which was designated micropapillomatosis and seems to be part of the metaplastic-neoplastic process [20−22]. The alteration is often seen in carcinoma in situ [22].

The next important pathogenetic step comprises cellular and epithelial atypia [16, 21−23, 26, 30, 38, 41, 47]. Cellular atypia in the bronchial epithelium usually occurs in

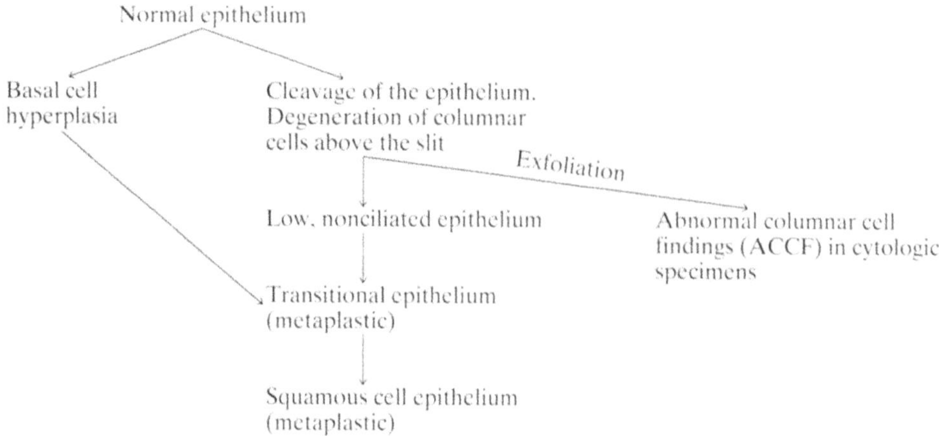

Fig. 6. Development of metaplastic epithelium in bronchial mucosa

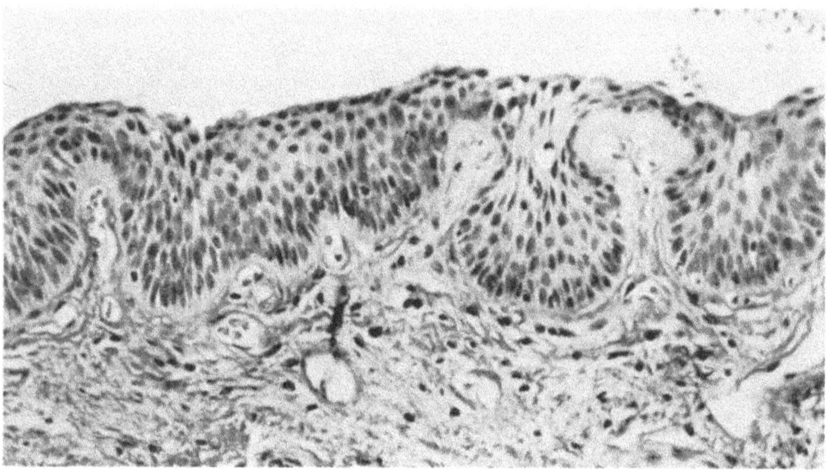

Fig. 7. Squamous metaplasia and micropapillomatosis. There are several protruding stroma papillae which are covered by a metaplastic epithelium. Van Gieson × 155

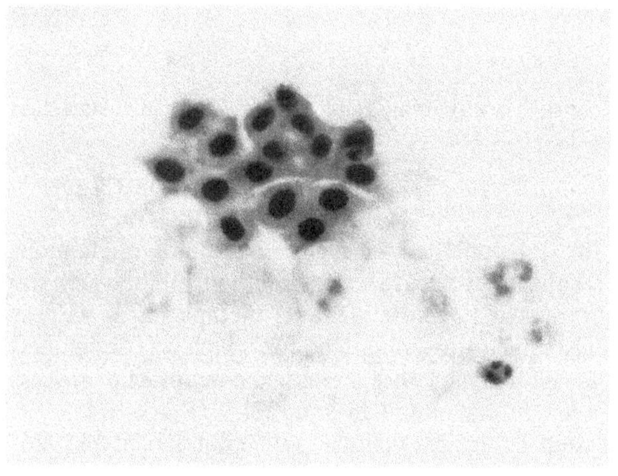

Fig. 8. Regular (non-atypical) squamous metaplastic cells. Sputum. Papanicolaou stain × 450

Table 1. Two hundred and eleven (211) consecutive cases with abnormal columnar cell findings (ACCF)

	Total material	No. cases with ACCF
Controls without metaplasia	328	33 (16%)
Controls with metaplasia	188	96 (45%)
Adenocarcinoma	22	6 (3%)
Squamous or undifferentiated carcinoma	137	76 (36%)
Total	675	211 (100%)

Adenocarcinoma and Squamous or undifferentiated carcinoma together: 39%

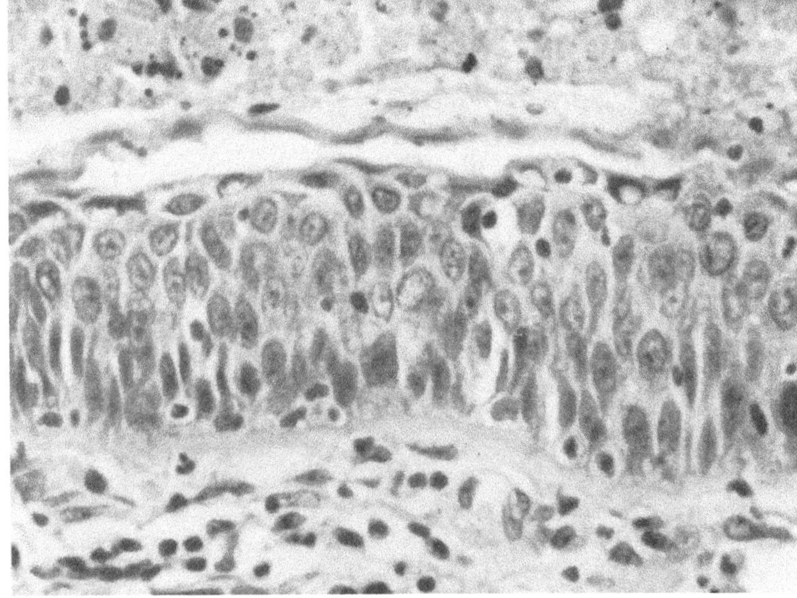

Fig. 9. Atypical metaplastic epithelium. The cells vary in size and shape. Most surface cells are elongated. The chromatin structure is variable. Hematoxylin-eosin × 250

metaplastically altered epithelium (Fig. 9) [16, 20, 21, 30, 37, 40, 48]. The atypia can be divided into mild, moderate, and severe (Fig. 1) [28, 36]. It may be difficult here as well as in cervical pathology to demarcate severe atypia from carcinoma in situ, which is the next step in the development.

The present studies as well as those of Saccomanno and Schreiber indicate that mild and also moderate epithelial atypia may be induced by noncarcinogenic agents [37, 40, 42, 43]. Severe atypia, however, can only be induced by carcinogenic substances in experimental systems [13].

The various degrees of atypia (mild, moderate, severe) in metaplastic epithelium can be identified cytologically (Figs. 10−12) and cytomorphologic criteria for these changes have been described [28, 30, 36, 37] (Table 2).

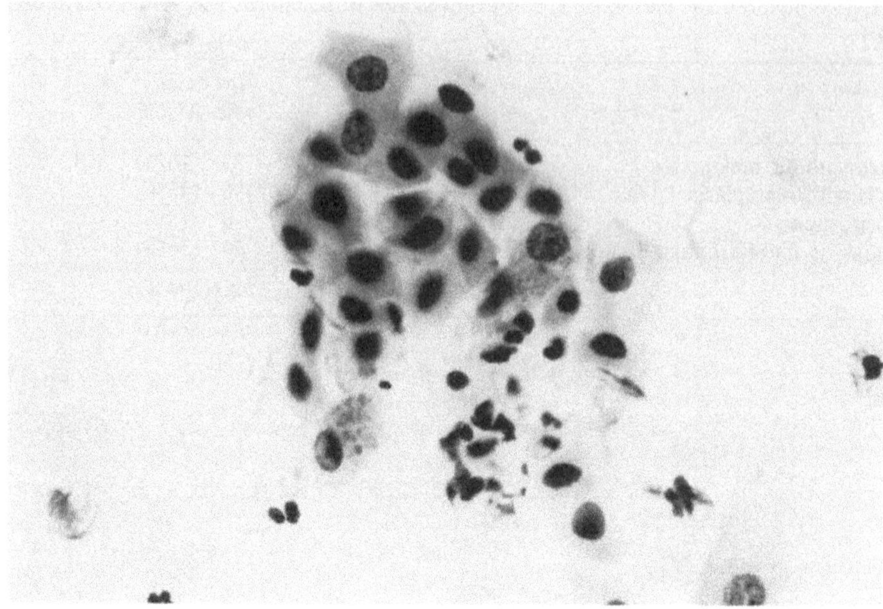

Fig. 10. Squamous metaplastic cells with mild atypia. Sputum. Papanicolaou stain × 250 [see also Table 2 and ref. 30]

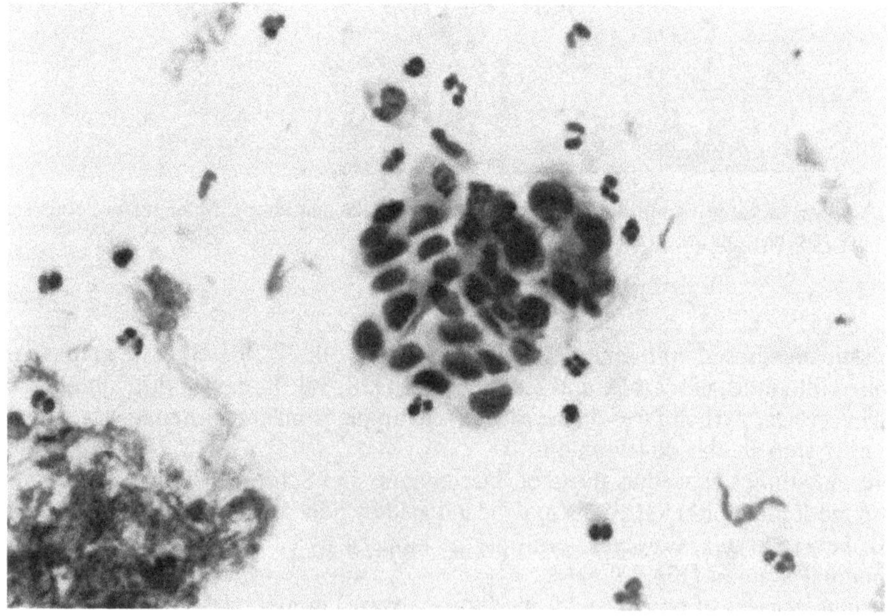

Fig. 11. Squamous metaplastic cells with moderate atypia. Sputum. Papanicolaou stain × 450 [see also Table 2 and ref. 30]

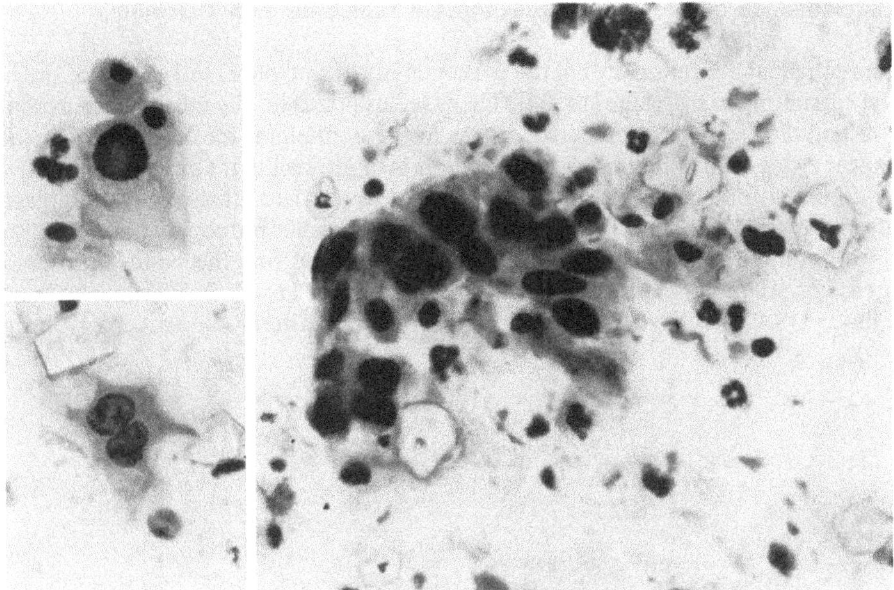

Fig. 12. Squamous metaplastic cells with severe atypia. Sputum. Papanicolaou stain × 450 [see also Table 2 and ref. 30]

Table 2. Grading of atypia in squamous metaplastic cells

Squamous metaplasia with:	Cell shape	Nuclear size and shape	Chromatin	Cell grouping
No atypia	Cubic, round, or slightly oval	Similar to that of oral squamous cells	Finely granular	Clusters[a]
Mild atypia	Slightly variable	Occasionally enlarged	Slight hyperchromasia in a few cells (finely granular)	Clusters[a]
Moderate atypia	Variable	Variable	Some nuclei show a distinct hyperchromasia (finely granular)	Clusters[a]; single cells may occur
Severe atypia	Distinct variation	Distinct variation	Nuclear hyperchromasia is striking in many cells (coarse chromatin)	Clusters[a] and/or single abnormal cells
Cancer cells (in situ and invasive carcinoma)	Marked variation	Marked variation	Hyperchromatic cells predominate (coarse chromatin)	Mainly single cells

[a] Of a metaplastic character (good cell adherence, flat surface, etc.)

Carcinoma In Situ — Early Bronchogenic Squamous Cell Carcinoma

The principal alteration during the pathogenesis of squamous cell cancer of the lung is the carcinoma in situ stage [14, 20]. There seems not to be any information available at present with respect to precursor stages in the epithelium for other histological lung cancer types than epidermoid carcinoma. It is of interest that epithelial atypias, which fulfill the criteria of carcinoma in situ, also occur almost exclusively in metaplastically altered epithelium (Fig. 13). This probably irreversible intraepithelial alteration can be differentiated cytologically from severe atypia on one the hand and outspoken invasive carcinoma on the other. In cooperation with Dr. L. B. Woolner at the Mayo Clinic, USA, we have set up cytomorphological criteria for very early bronchial

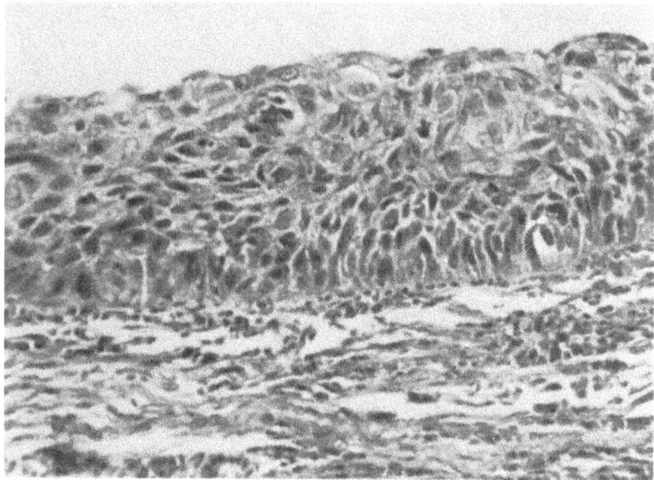

Fig. 13. Carcinoma in situ in the bronchial mucosa, Van Gieson × 250

Table 3. Cytologic findings in carcinoma in situ with or without early stromal invasion

1) Epidermoid carcinoma cells, mainly occurring singly, with a less bizarre appearance than cells representing outspoken invasive squamous cell carcinoma

2) Large, polygonal, round or irregular cells with abundant orangeophilic or eosinophilic cytoplasm and large, slightly hyperchromatic nuclei

3) Small abnormal keratinized squamous cells, usually round or oval

4) Absence of tumor diathesis

Table 4. Carcinoma in situ with early stromal invasion in clinically occult and early bronchogenic carcinoma (epidermoid)

No. of patients	57
Positive cytology	53
Positive bronchoscopic biopsy	26
Histological evidence of early stromal invasion	39 (68%)

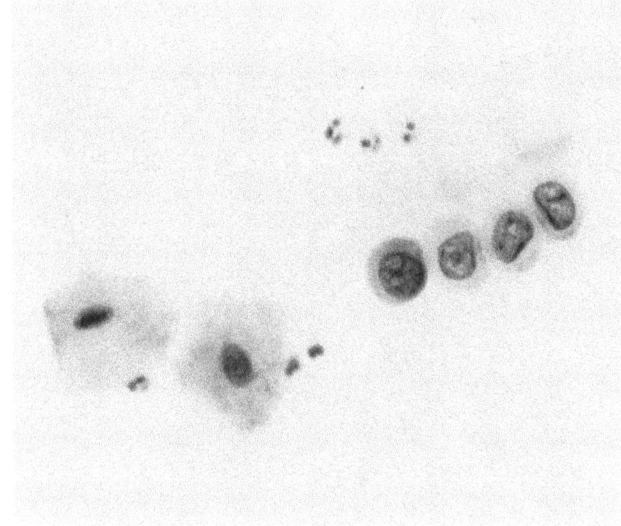

Fig. 14. Four small, round or cubic, keratinized cancer cells from a proven case of bronchogenic carcinoma in situ with early stromal invasion. There are two oral squamous cells to the left. Sputum. Papanicolaou stain × 450

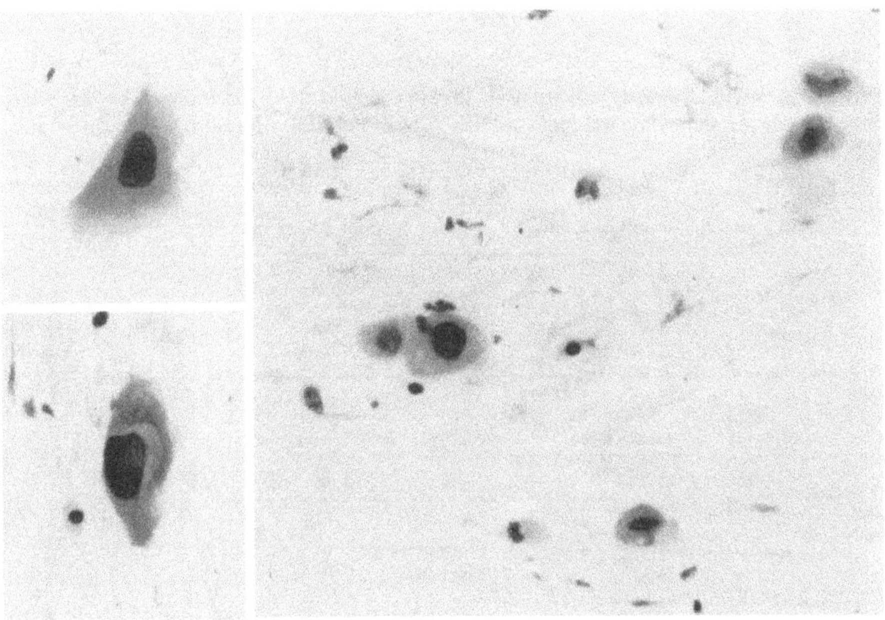

Fig. 15. Some polygonal and slightly irregular keratinized cancer cells with abundant cytoplasm from a proven case of carcinoma in situ. Sputum. Papanicolaou stain × 450

carcinoma, i.e., carcinoma in situ with or without early stromal invasion (Figs. 14, 15) [28, 30, 36].

The relationship between cancer in situ and invasive carcinoma is emphasized by the fact that early invasive features were observed in 68% of 57 cases of early lung cancer after semiserial sectioning of surgical material from cases which showed carcinoma in situ lesions at primary examination of bronchoscopic biopsies [27] (Table 4). The fact

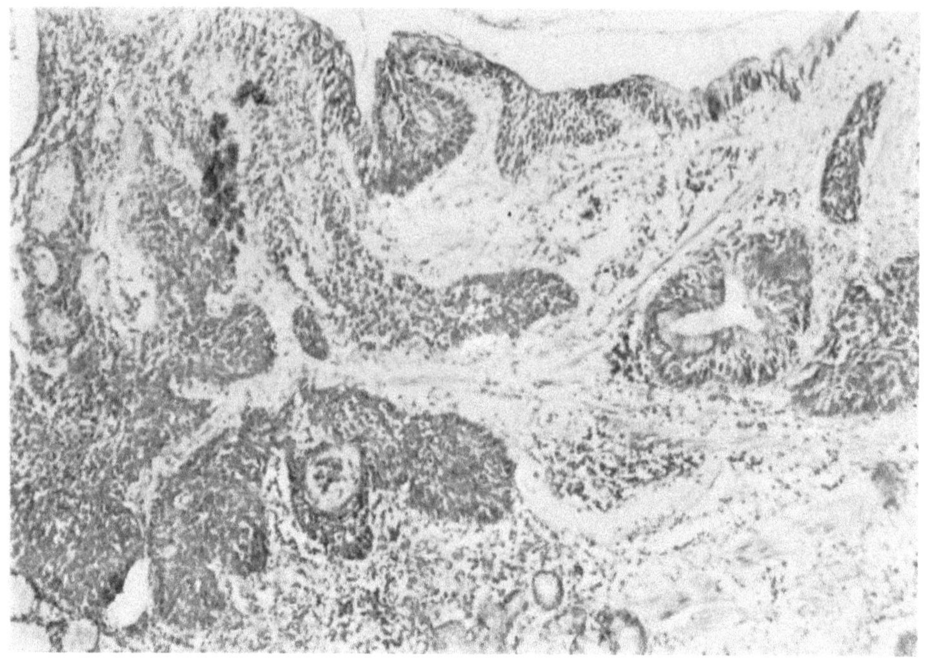

Fig. 16. A small, radically exstirpated, invasive epidermoid carcinoma. At the edge of the invasive cancer there is carcinoma in situ *(upper middle)*. Hematoxylin-eosin × 100

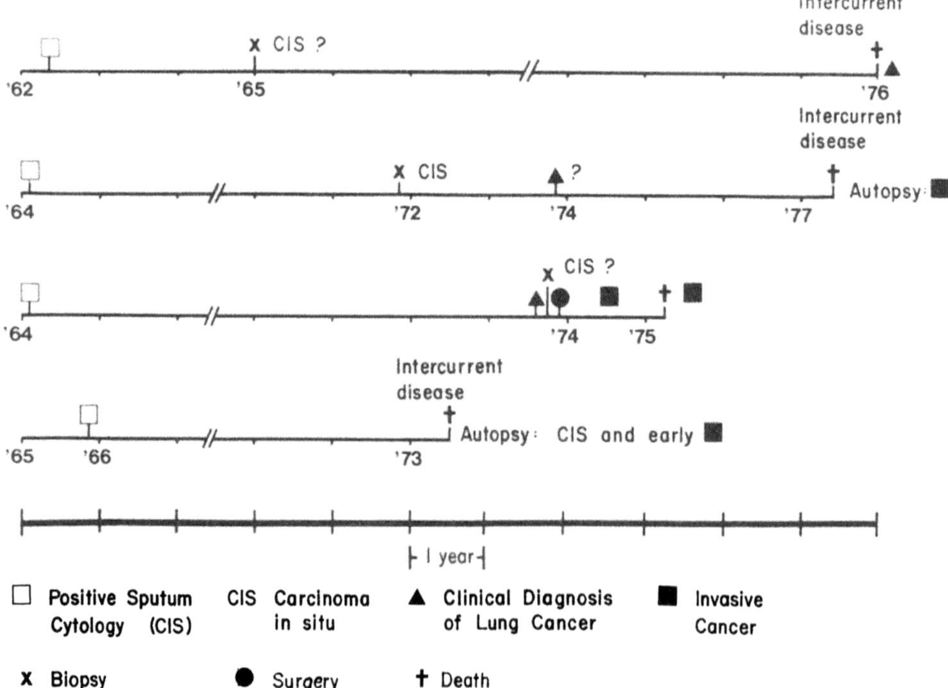

Fig. 17. Bronchogenic squamous cell carcinoma. Cytological evidence of long preclinical evolution

that carcinoma in situ may be observed at the edge of an early but unquestionably invasive squamous cell cancer further supports the assumption that invasive squamous cell lung cancer usually is preceded by an in situ lesion. Several such lesions have been observed in the Sabbatsberg Hospital study of "asymptomatic" cigarette smokers, who were screened for early detection of lung cancer and "premalignant" changes by sputum cytology (Fig. 16) [5, 29, 44].

This material of cigarette smokers contains, in addtion, several cases with a long preclinical stage similar to that of early cervix cancer (cancer in situ) [14]. Figure 17 illustrates some clinically occult cases which for several years displayed squamous cancer cells in their sputa indicative of early or in situ squamous cell carcinoma [5, 29]. These cases revealed clinical or histological evidence of invasive carcinoma after a clinically occult period of 8–14 years from the first positive sputum examination [14, 29, 44].

Quantitative Cytochemical Studies:
Sequential Occurrence of Abnormal Bronchial Cells in an Experimental System

Some cytochemical studies were performed in order to test whether there is a sequence of changes in the bronchial epithelium which can be identified by sputum cytology and which possesses cytochemical qualities that indicate the existence of a progressive and gradual malignant transformation to invasive lung cancer. The first studies were performed on human sputum material [1, 30]. It was found that parallel with an increasing degree of cellular atypia in squamous metaplastic epithelium there is an increasing degree of aneuploidy (heteroploidy; Fig. 18). These cytological and cytochemical changes indicate that progressive cellular events occur during the pathogenesis of bronchogenic carcinoma.

The conclusions which are based on studies on human sputum material from various individuals are supported by experiments on beagle dogs in which the progress of changes has been followed in the same individual (dog). These ongoing experiments are performed in cooperation with Professor Hayata's lung cancer study group at Tokyo Medical College Hospital. 20-Methylcholanthrene is injected in the submucosa at a well-defined locus in the bronchial tree. By means of bronchofiberscope, brush cell samples are regularly obtained and analyzed by cytomorphological grading and quantitative cytochemical techniques [11].

The DNA distribution pattern of normal columnar cells, non-atypical (regular) squamous metaplastic cells, metaplastic cells with various degrees of nuclear atypia, and finally cancer cells was studied in the brush samples. It was found that regular metaplastic cells exhibited normal diploid DNA values. Cells with mild atypia had DNA values within the normal 2C–4C region, whereas metaplastic cells with moderate atypia, severe atypia, and cancer cells exhibited DNA values exceeding the normal 4C region, together with progressively scattered DNA values [11, 13]. It was concluded that regular exposure of bronchial epithelium in beagle dogs to 20-methylcholanthrene induces progressive cytochemical and morphological alterations in the epithelium which finally develop into carcinoma.

As part of this experiment on dogs, the relative numbers of squamous metaplastic cells with various degrees of atypia and squamous cancer cells occurring in the bronchial smear preparations at different periods after the beginning of the experiment were studied. During the continued treatment, cells with more pronounced atypia and

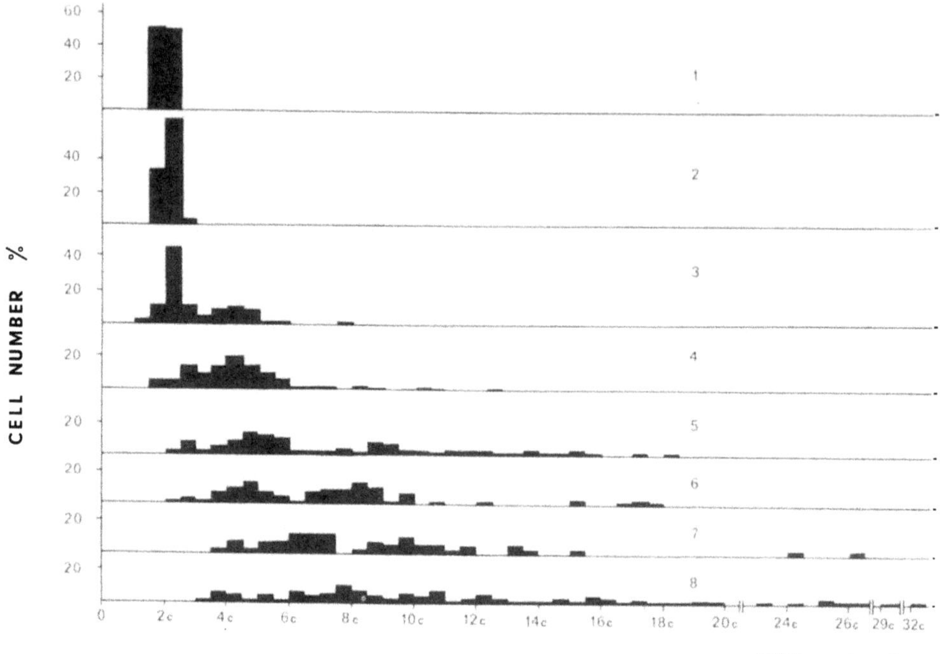

Fig. 18. Mean amount of DNA (Feulgen stain) in atypical squamous metaplastic and neoplastic bronchial epithelial cells. *1*, Control cells (leukocytes). *2*, Regular squamous metaplastic cells. *3*, Metaplastic cells with mild nuclear atypia. *4*, Metaplastic cells with moderate atypia. *5*, Metaplastic cells with severe atypia. *6*, Squamous metaplastic cells with borderline atypia (to carcinoma in situ). *7*, Carcinoma in situ. *8*, Invasive carcinoma

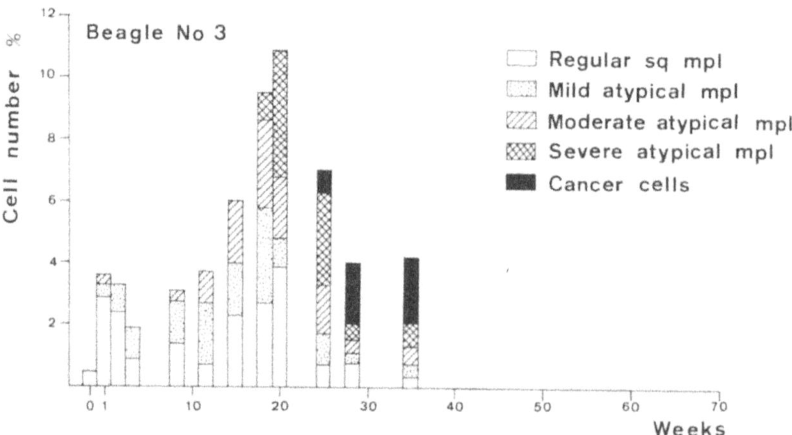

Fig. 19. Percentage of regular squamous metaplastic cells, metaplastic cells with various degrees of nuclear atypia, and cancer cells in a beagle dog which was treated for 35 weeks. 20-Methylcholanthrene was injected in the submucosa at the bifurcation of the apical and cardiac bronchi

cancer cells were found. A progressive increase of cells with more pronounced atypia could be observed throughout the experiment. Figure 19 shows the cell distribution in one of the dogs. The distribution of abnormal cells was similar in the other dogs [13].

"Cigarette Cancer" Pathogenesis: A Two-Step Process?

It is possible that a relationship exists between an early epithelial injury (slit formation – ACCF) and the effect of certain components in cigarette smoke. According to studies by Hammond et al. [6], it is possible that the benzpyrene in cigarettes alone does not produce lung cancer. It is well known, however, that heavy cigarette smoking produces a high lung cancer risk. It is of considerable interest to note that it has been possible to produce lung cancer experimentally almost only when the carcinogen, usually benzpyrene, has been combined with damage of the mucociliary apparatus [2].

Various substances in the cigarette smoke may have different effects on the respiratory epithelium [31, 32]. It seems possible that slit formation (Figs. 2, 3) and expulsion or exfoliation of abundant columnar epithelium (ACCF; Fig. 5) resulting in a low nonciliated epithelium (Fig. 4) may be the result of the action of onrspecific irritants of the cigarette smoke, i.e., hydrogen cyanide, acrolein, formaldehyde, and nitrogen oxides [2, 7, 50]. This would be the first step in a two-step process, which may lead to lung cancer [2]. The unprotected low nonciliated epithelium develops squamous metaplasia as a protective reaction. The low epithelium and presumably also the metaplastic epithelium is probably sensitive to the action of carcinogenic substances as the mucociliary protecting mechanism is injured [8, 9]. The second step in the process would imply that benzpyrene, possibly under the influence of the hereditary enzyme aryl hydrocarbon hydroxylase (AHH), produces a potent carcinogenic metabolite (epoxide) [4, 12]. Benzpyrene or its metabolites induce atypia, which increases in degree up to carcinoma in situ, which may develop into invasive carcinoma (Fig. 20). This theory is supported by several studies [10, 15, 18]. Other authors have, however, reached deviating conclusions with respect to the importance of AHH [19, 33].

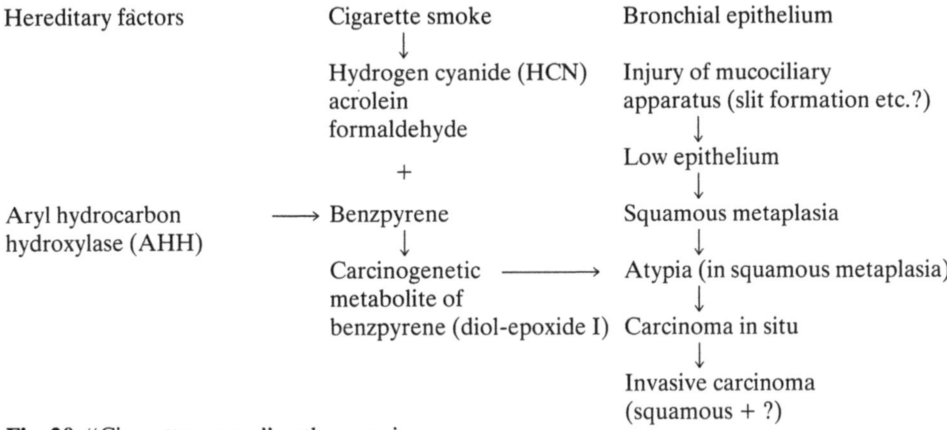

Fig. 20. "Cigarette cancer" pathogenesis

M. Nasiell et al.

Conclusions

The observations and results indicate that squamous cell bronchial cancer develops stepwise over a long period (10–20 years or more) with a series of alterations in the bronchial mucosa. These sequential changes can be identified cytologically, which is of great importance for clinical and experimental studies of the pathogenesis of epidermoid lung cancer.

A progressive increase and variation in nuclear DNA content occurs parallel to an increasing degree of cellular and nuclear atypia. Carcinoma in situ (with or without early stromal invasion) is a histocytological entity of prime importance for the early diagnosis of epidermoid lung cancer, and for the understanding of the pathogenetic process. It seems further possible that the process is composed of two or several principally different stages. Certain gaseous components of the cigarette smoke produce an epithelial injury, i.e., the mucociliary apparatus is damaged. This makes the next step possible, in which metabolites of benzpyrene produce the neoplastic process, demonstrated morphologically and cytochemically by increasing epithelial atypia and DNA abnormalities, which finally results in carcinoma.

References

1. Auer G, Kato H, Nasiell M, Roger V, Zetterberg A, Karlen L (1980) Cytophotometric DNA-analysis of atypical squamous metaplastic cells, carcinoma in situ, and bronchogenic carcinoma. In: Nieburgs HE (ed) Prevention and detection of cancer, vol. 2/II. Marcel Dekker, New York Basel, pp 1467–1976
2. Carlens E (1979) Smoking and occupation. In: Ramstrom L (ed) The smoking epidemic. Fourth World Conference on Smoking and Health. Almqvist & Wiksell, Stockholm, pp 54–56
3. Frost JK, Gupta PK, Erozan YS et al. (1973) Pulmonary cytologic alterations in toxic environmental inhalation. Hum Pathol 4:521–536
4. Gelboin HV (1972) Mechanisms of induction of drug metabolism enzymes. In: La Du BN, Mandel HG, Leong-Way E (eds) Fundamentals of drug metabolism and drug disposition. Williams and Wilkins, Baltimore, pp 279–307
5. Haglund S, Kinnman J, Malström L, Nasiell K, Nasiell M, Roger V (1979) The Sabbatsberg Hospital sputum cytologic study of roentgenologically occult bronchial cancer (in Swedish). Lakartidningen 76:735–738
6. Hammond EC, Selikoff IJ, Lawther PL, Seidman H (1976) Inhalation of benzpyrene and cancer in man. Ann NY Acad Sci 271:116–124
7. Higenbottam T, Clark TJH, Shipley MJ, Rose G (1980) Lung function and symptoms of cigarette smokers related to tar yield and number of cigarettes smoked. Lancet 1:409–412
8. Hilding AC (1956a) On cigarette smoking, bronchial carcinoma and ciliary action. III. Accumulation of cigarette tar upon artificially produced deciliated islands in the respiratory epithelium. Ann Otol 65:116–130
9. Hilding AC (1956b) On smoking, bronchial carcinoma and ciliary action. N Engl J Med 254:1155–1160
10. Ho W, Wilcox K, Furst A (1974) Pulmonary carcinogenesis by two aryl hydrocarbons on three mouse strains. In: Karbe E, Park JF (eds) Experimental lung cancer. Carcinogenesis and bioassays. Springer, Berlin Heidelberg New York, pp 62–71
11. Kato H, Saito T, Iimura I et al. (1980) Studies of the carcinogenetic process of experimental pulmonary squamous carcinoma and the clinical applications. Jpn J Lung Cancer 20:49–58

12. Kellermann GH, Shaw CF, Luyten-Kellermann M (1973) Aryl hydrocarbon hydroxylase inducibility and bronchogenic carcinoma. N Engl J Med 289:934–937
13. Konaka C, Auer G, Nasiell M et al. (to be published) Pathogenesis of squamous bronchial carcinoma in 20-methylcholanthrene treated beagle dogs. Anal Quant Cytol
14. Koss LG (1979) Diagnostic cytology and its histopathologic bases, 3rd edn. J. B. Lippincott, Philadelphia Toronto
15. Kouri RE, Demoise CF, Whitmire CE (1974) The significance or aryl hydrocarbon hydroxylase enzyme systems in the selection of model systems for respiratory carcinogenesis. In: Karbe E, Park JF (eds) Experimental lung cancers. Carcinogenesis and bioassays. Springer, Berlin Heidelberg New York, pp 48–61
16. McDowell EM, Becci PJ, Barrett LA, Trump BF (1978) Morphogenesis and classification of lung cancer. In: Harris CC (ed) Pathogenesis and therapy of lung cancer. Marcel Dekker, New York Basel, pp 445–519
17. Melamed MR, Zaman MB, Flehinger BJ, Martini N (1977) Radiologically occult in situ and incipient invasive epidermoid lung cancer. Detection by sputum cytology in a survey of asymptomatic cigarette smokers. Am J Surg Pathol 1:5–16
18. Mohr U, Reznik G (1978) Tobacco carcinogenesis. In: Harris CC (ed) Pathogenesis and therapy of lung cancer. Marcel Dekker, New York Basel, pp 263–367
19. Mulvihill JJ (1978) Host factors. In: Harris CC (ed) Pathogenesis and therapy of lung cancer. Marcel Dekker, New York Basel, pp 53–71
20. Müller K-M (1979a) Morphologie und Häufigkeit präinvasiver Neoplasien und früher Carcinome. In: Georgii A (Hrsg) Frühe Tumoren in Diagnostik und Therapie. Verh Dtsch Krebs-Ges, Bd 2. Fisher, Stuttgart New York
21. Müller K-M (1979b) Krebsvorstadien der Bronchialschleimhaut. Verh Dtsch Ges Pathol 63:112–131
22. Nasiell M (1963) The general appearance of the bronchial epithelium in bronchial carcinoma: a histopathological udy with some cytological viewpoints. Acta Cytol (Baltimore) 7:97–106
23. Nasiell M (1966) Metaplasia ana atypical metaplasia in the bronchial epithelium. A histopathologic and cytopathologic study. Acta Cytol (Baltimore) 10:421–427
24. Nasiell M (1967) Abnormal columnar cell findings in bronchial epithelium. A cytologic and histologic study of lung cancer and non-cancer cases. Acta Cytol (Baltimore) 11:397–402
25. Nasiell M (1968a) Comparative histological and sputumcytological studies of the bronchial epithelium in inflammatory and neoplastic lung disease. Acta Pathol Microbiol Scand 72:501–518
26. Nasiell M (1968b) Sputumcytologic changes in smokers and nonsmokers in relation to chronic inflammatory lung diseases. Acta Pathol Microbiol Scand 74:205–213
27. Nasiell M (1969) Early cancer of the lung. In: Royal Society of Health, London: International Health Conference 1968: addresses and papers. Oscar Blackford, London Truro, pp 23–29
28. Nasiell M (1976) Cytology of benign changes and carcinoma in situ of the lung. In: Wied GL, Koss LG, Reagan JW (eds) Tutorial proceedings of the International Academy of Cytology: compendium on diagnostic cytology, vol IV, 4th edn. Tutorials of Cytology, Chicago, pp 315–329
29. Nasiell M, Sinner W, Tornvall G (1977) Clinically occult lung cancer with positive sputum cytology and primarily negative roentgenologic findings. Scand J Respir Dis 58:134–144
30. Nasiell M, Kato H, Auer G, Zetterberg A, Roger V, Karlen L (1978) Cytomorphological grading and Feulgen DNA-analysis of metaplastic and neoplastic bronchial cells. Cancer 41:1511–1521
31. Nettesheim P (1974) Review and introductory remarks: multifactorial respiratory carcinogenesis. In: Karbe E, Park JF (eds) Experimental lung cancer; carcinogenesis and bioassays. Springer Berlin Heidelberg New York, pp 157–172

32. Nettesheim P, Griesemer R (1978) Experimental models for studies of respiratory tract carcinogenesis. In: Harris CC (ed) Pathogenesis and therapy of lung cancer. Marcel Dekker, New York Basel, pp 75–188
33. Paigen B, Gurtoo HL, Minowada J et al. (1977) Questionable relation of aryl hydrocarbon hydroxylase to lung cancer risk. N Engl J Med 297: 346–350
34. Papanicolaou GN, Bridges EL, Railey C (1961) Degeneration of the ciliated cells of the bronchial epithelium (ciliocytophthoria) in its relation to pulmonary disease. Am Rev Respir Dis 83: 641–659
35. Plamenac P, Nikulin A, Kahvic M (1970) Cytology of the respiratory tract in advanced age. Acta Cytol (Baltimore) 14: 526–530
36. Riotton G, Christopherson WM, Lunt R (eds) (1977) Cytology of non-gynaecological sites, 17. International Histological Classification of Tumours. World Health Organization, Geneva
37. Saccomanno G (1978) Diagnostic pulmonary cytology. Am Soc Clin Pathol, Chicago
38. Saccomanno G, Saunders RP, Archer VE, Auerbach O, Kuschner M, Beckler PA (1965) Cancer of the lung: the cytology of sputum prior to the development of carcinoma. Acta Cytol (Baltimore) 9: 413–423
39. Saccomanno G, Archer VE, Auerbach O, Saunders RP, Brennan LM (1974) Development of carcinoma of the lung as reflected in exfoliated cells. Cancer 33: 356–370
40. Schreiber H (1978) Cytopathology. In: Harris CC (ed) Pathogenesis and therapy of lung cancer. Marcel Dekker, New York and Basel, pp 521–557
41. Schreiber H, Saccomanno G, Martin DH, Brennan L (1974) Sequential cytological changes during development of respiratory tract tumors induced in hamsters by benzo(a)pyrene-ferric oxide. Cancer Res 34: 689–698
42. Schreiber H, Bibbo M, Wied GL, Saccomanno G, Nettesheim P (1979) Bronchial metaplasia as a benign or premalignant lesion. I. Cytologic and ultrastructural discrimination between acute carcinogen effects and toxin-induced changes. Acta Cytol (Baltimore) 23: 496–503
43. Schreiber H, Bibbo M, Wied GL, Saccomanno G, Nettesheim P (to be published) Bronchial metaplasia as a benign or premalignant lesion. II. Cytologic discrimination of persistent or progressive carcinogen effects. Acta Cytol (Baltimore)
44. Sinner WN, Nasiell M, Tornvall G (1977) Primär Roentgennegativer Lungenkrebs bei Positiver Sputumzytologie. Fortschr Roentgenstr 127: 507–513
45. Stenbäck F (1973) Morphologic characteristics of experimentally induced lung tumors and their precursors in hamsters. Acta Cytol (Baltimore) 17: 476–486
46. Stenbäck F (1977) Morphology of experimentally induced respiratory tumors in syrian golden hamster. A histological, histochemical and ultrastructural study. Acta Otolaryngol [Suppl] (Stockh) 347: 1–59
47. Suprun H, Hjerpe A, Nasiell M, Vogel B (1980) A correlative cytologic study on the incidence of pulmonary cancer and other lung diseases associated with squamous metaplasia of the bronchial epithelium. In: Nieburgs HE (ed) Prevention and detection of cancer, vol 2/II. Marcel Dekker, New York Basel, pp 1477–1483
48. Trump BF, McDowell EM, Glavin F et al. (1978) The respiratory epithelium. III. Histogenesis of epidermoid metaplasia and carcinoma in situ in the human. J Natl Cancer Inst 61: 563–575
49. Vassilakos P (1976) Cytopathologie des cancers broncho-pulmonaires. Huber, Berne Stuttgart Vienna
50. Walker TR, Kiefer JE (1966) Ciliastic components in the gas phase of cigarette smoke. Science 153: 1248–1250

Lung Cancer Histogenesis Following in Vivo Bronchial Injections of 20-Methylcholanthrene in Dogs

H. Kato, C. Konaka, Y. Hayata, J. Ono, I. Iimura,
Y. Matsushima, M. Tahara, J. Lei, M. Nasiell, and G. Auer

Tokyo Medical College Hospital, Department of Surgery, 6-7-1 Nishishinjuku,
Shinjuku-ku, Tokyo 160, Japan

Introduction

The therapeutic results of lung cancer have not improved much during the last decade despite increasing incidence throughout the world. If the disease could be detected at an early stage, improved therapeutic results could be expected.

Clarification of the carcinogenic process of bronchogenic carcinoma might demonstrate characteristic precancerous changes and improve early cancer detection and therapeutic results. Such information might furthermore lead to progress in the prevention of lung cancer.

After studying the carcinogenic process of pulmonary squamous cell carcinoma, some investigators have found evidence that atypical squamous metaplasia may be a significant stage in the carcinogenic process [1–3, 22–24, 28, 29, 31, 34], but others [15, 32] have contended that the carcinogenic process does not involve cellular transformation to cancer from squamous metaplasia passing through a sequential progression of nuclear atypia.

Nakajima [19] produced peripheral lung cancers in dogs with a high success rate by means of 20-methylcholanthrene (20-MC) instilled via a vinyl catheter inserted deeply into the lower lobe bronchi. This method required, however, approximately 3 years for the development of the carcinomas. Recently the present authors [9, 10] succeeded in producing central-type lung cancer in the large bronchi of dogs within a relatively short period by injections of the same carcinogen into the bronchial submucosa, and studied the changes in the bronchial epithelium during the carcinogenic process by fiberoptic bronchoscopy and by cytological, histological, and cytochemical analyses.

Materials and Methods

The experiments included four adult beagles and six mongrels. 20-Methylcholanthrene was used as carcinogen (Sigma Co., USA). The diet was ordinary dog food (Oriental Kobo Co., Tokyo).

The flexible needle (Fig. 1) for the injection of 20-MC through the fiberoptic bronchoscope (Olympus BF-IT) was developed by the authors. It is now commercially available as the Olympus NM-1D. General anesthesia was performed by intravenous injection of Isozol (thiamital sodium).

Recent Results in Cancer Research, Vol. 82
© Springer-Verlag Berlin · Heidelberg 1982

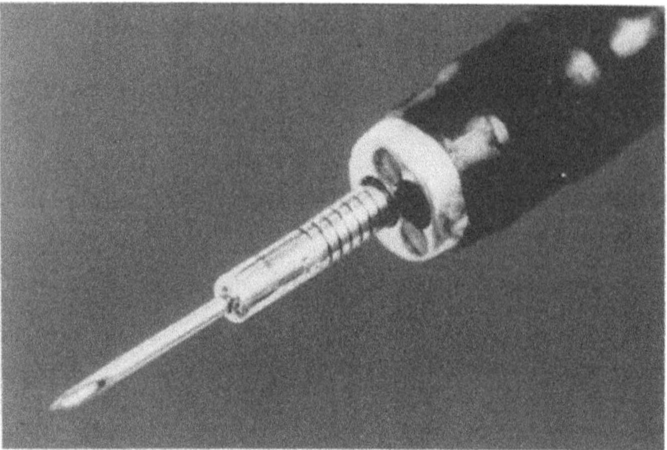

Fig. 1. Needle designed for use via the fiberoptic bronchoscope. The length of the entire instrument with the tip extended is 11.5 cm, the retractable tip is 0.8 cm in length and 1.4 mm in diameter. It can be passed through the instrumentation channel of Olympus 1T fiberoptic bronchoscope

The dogs were divided into three experimental groups. The first group, consisting of two beagles and four mongrels, were given injections of 50 g 20-MC dissolved in 1.5 ml distilled water into the submucosa of the bifurcation of the apical and cardiac lobe bronchi every week. Fiberoptic bronchoscopic observation and brushing for cytology were performed once a week prior to the injection of 20-MC. Biopsy for histological examination was performed monthly.

In the second group, which included one beagle and one mongrel, only a single injection of 50 mg 20-MC was given in the same locus as in the first group. The bronchial epithelium was examined cytologically after 1, 2, and 4 days, and thereafter every 7 days, up to 7 months after the injection.

The third group, which also consisted of one beagle and one mongrel, were given weekly injections of 1.5 ml of sterile water. The bronchial epithelium was examined in the same way as in the second group.

Brush specimens for cytological evaluation from the pertinent loci were smeared on glass slides and fixed immediately with isopropyl alcohol and stained according to Papanicolaou's method. The biopsy specimens were fixed in 10% formalin and stained with hematoxylin-eosin.

Histomorphology

The histomorphology of the bronchial mucosa comprising normal and altered epithelium exhibits great similarity to the respiratory mucosa in man as shown in Figs. 2, 4−8 [16, 17, 20, 21, 29]. The grading of epithelial atypia is based on previous studies on human bronchial material [21, 28, 29].

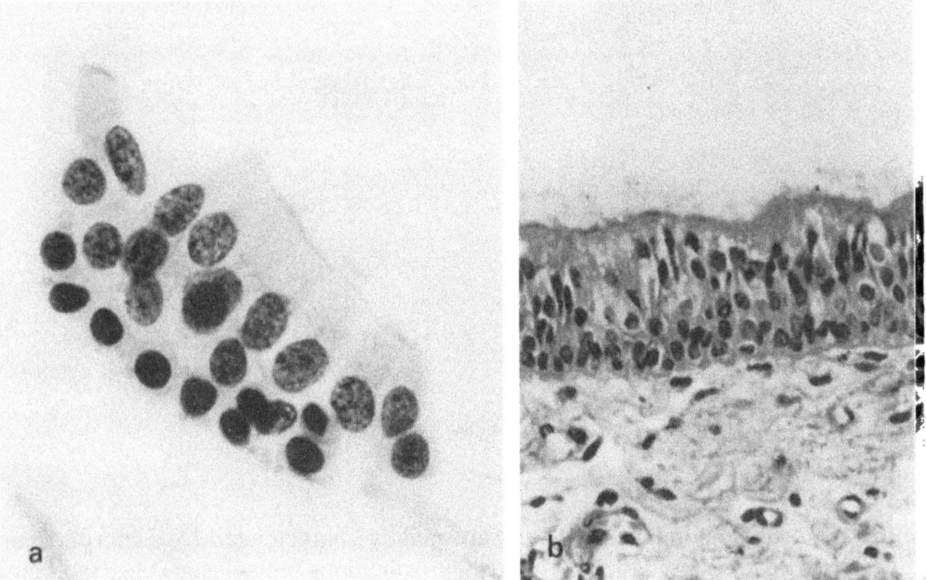

Fig. 2a, b. Normal dog bronchial epithelium. **a** Brush cytology (× 400). **b** Biopsy histology (× 100)

Cytomorphology

The cytomorphology of normal and altered bronchial cells also shows great similarity to corresponding findings in human cytologic material [23, 29]. The minor deviations are included below in the detailed description of the various cellular changes.

Normal Columnar Epithelium

Figure 2 illustrates ordinary respiratory columnar cells in a beagle dog.

Basal Cell Hyperplasia

Basal cells are easily recognized in the brush materials. Basal cells are round with relatively large nuclear/cytoplasmic (N/C) ratio. The cells occur in clusters with good cellular adherence. The definition of basal cell hyperplasia is based on the occurrence of clusters comprising numerous basal cells, usually in a well preserved monolayer arrangement. This phenomenon is now being further investigated in brush material.

Atypical basal cell hyperplasia is mainly characterized by the occurrence of prominent nucleoli and a slightly increased and variable nuclear size (Fig. 12).

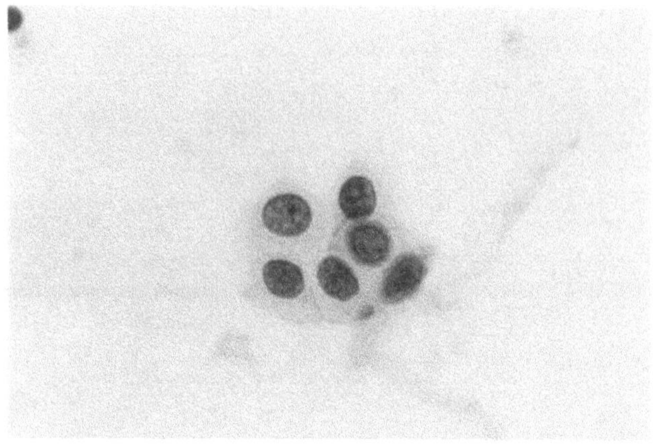

Fig. 3. Regular squamous metaplastic cells of mongrel C5, one week after injection. Brush cytology (× 400)

Immature Squamous Metaplasia

Immature squamous metaplastic cells are mainly characterized by a morphological appearance corresponding to that of regular squamous metaplastic cells (see below) with the exception that the cytoplasm lacks any sign of keratinization when studied by means of the Papanicolaou staining technique.

Regular Metaplastic Cells

Cells occur mainly in clusters. There is good cell adherence with only occasional single metaplastic cells. There is often a flat surface in the metaplastic cell cluster indicating bronchial mucosa origin. The metaplastic cells are smaller than oral squamous cells and larger than basal cells. The cell shape is polygonal, cuboidal, or spherical and in Papanicolaou stained preparations the cytoplasm is usually cyanophilic (basophilic) or light green. The nuclear chromatin is finely granular and prominent nucleoli are not present (Fig. 3).

Metaplastic Cells with Mild Atypia

Cell und nuclear size are slightly variable. The nuclear chromatin is finely granular or more distinctly granular. There is usually no hyperchromasia. A small nucleolus may be seen. The cytoplasm is usually cyanophilic or light green. Single cells are rare (Fig. 4).

Metaplastic Cells with Moderate Atypia

Cell and nuclear size are variable. Multinucleation may occur. The nuclei are usually larger than those of non-atypical and mildly atypical cells. Slight hyperchromasia is common with a distinct nuclear membrane and distinct nucleoli. The cytoplasm is cyanophilic or light green or occasionally eosinophilic. Single metaplastic cells may occur (Fig. 5).

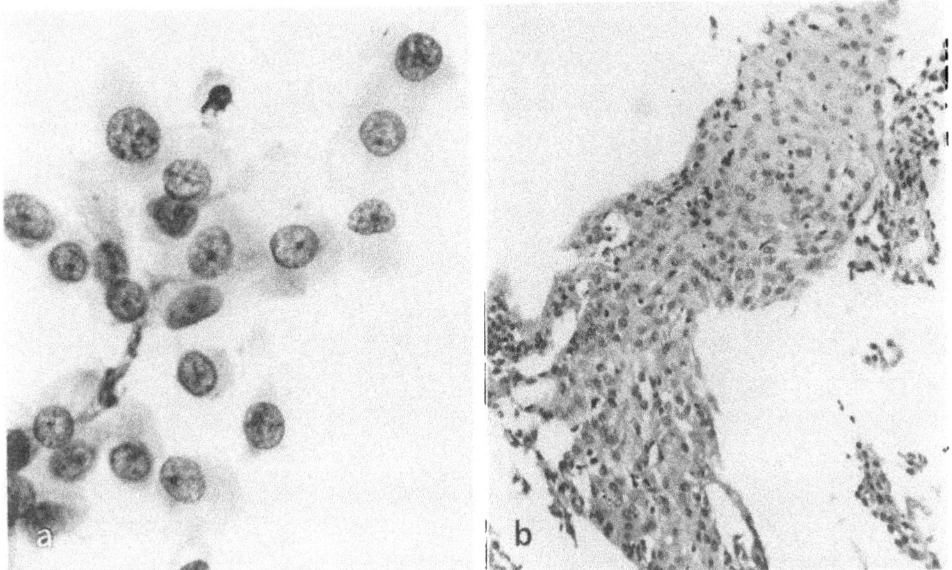

Fig. 4a, b. Mild atypical immature or squamous metaplasia of beagle B5 after 2 weeks. Note slight variation in nuclear size. **a** Brush cytology (× 400). **b** Biopsy histology (× 100)

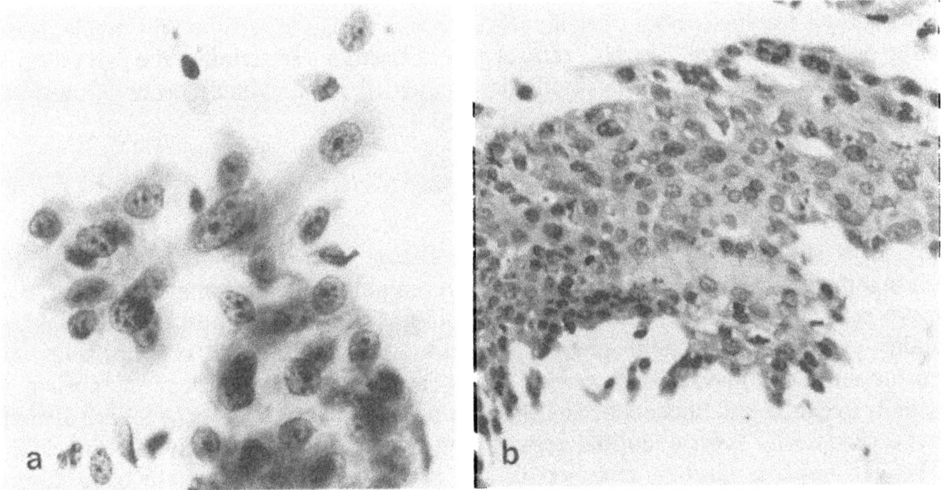

Fig. 5a, b. Moderate atypical immature metaplasia of beagle B5 after 3 weeks. Hyperchromasia, variation of nuclear size, and prominent nucleoli are seen. **a** Brush cytology (× 400). **b** Biopsy histology (× 150)

Metaplastic Cells with Severe Atypia

The cells still occur in clusters and show a pavement-like arrangement. Cellular overlapping is common. There is a distinct variation in cellular and nuclear size and shape. Nuclear hyperchromasia is present but not as pronounced as in corresponding

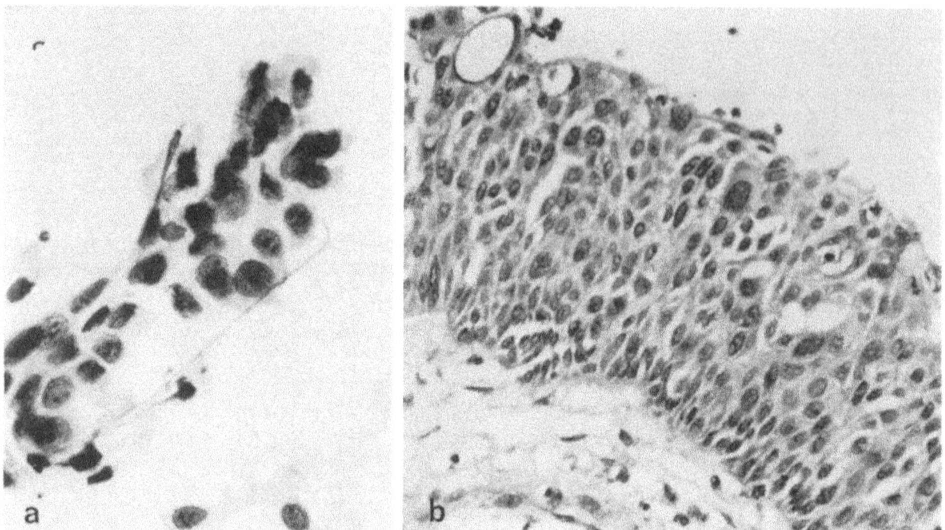

Fig. 6a, b. Severe immature metaplasia of mongrel C3 after 11 weeks. Hyperchromasia, striking variation of nuclear size, and prominent nucleoli are demonstrated. **a** Brush cytology (× 400). **b** Biopsy histology (× 200)

human cell types. The nuclear membrane may be irregular and thickened and the chromatin is usually coarse. Prominent, sometimes irregular, eosinophilic nucleoli are often a striking feature. The N/C ratio is generally large. On staining, the cytoplasm is cyanophilic, light green, or eosinophilic. Though the cells mainly occur in clusters, single atypical metaplastic cells are frequent (Fig. 6).

Carcinoma in Situ

The cells still occur in clusters, but single cancer cells are frequent. The cellular arrangement is pavementlike with distinct overlapping. The abnormal cell clusters are more cellular than in severe atypical metaplasia. The cytoplasm in the cell clusters stains cyanophilic or light green. The abnormal single cells often display an eosinophilic cytoplasm. The nuclear shape is variable. The nuclear membrane is usually irregular and thickened. The chromatin is granular or coarse. There is a distinct hyperchromasia. Most abnormal cells exhibit irregular and relatively large nucleoli. The N/C ratio is large. Carcinoma in situ is difficult to differentiate from severe atypical metaplasia in cytologic brush specimens and histology is needed for definitive diagnosis (Fig. 7).

Invasive Carcinoma

Large single cells occur with striking nuclear abnormalities. However, the abnormal cells still also occur in loose groups with weak cellular adherence. A coarsely granular chromatin, striking hyperchromasia, irregular and thickened nuclear membranes, and large abnormal nucleoli are seen. These cellular features are more pronounced than in severe atypical metaplasia and carcinoma in situ (Fig. 8).

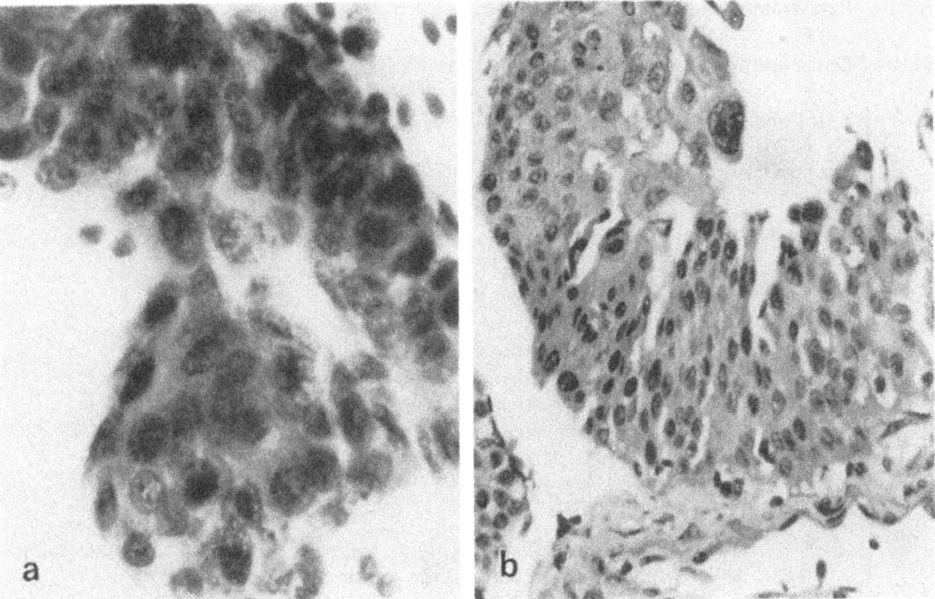

Fig. 7a, b. Carcinoma in situ of beagle B6 after 18 weeks. Distinct overlapping of cells, hyperchromasia, and coarse chromatin are seen. Carcinoma in situ is difficult to differentiate cytologically from severe atypical metaplasia. The definite diagnosis was made by histology. **a** Brush cytology (× 400). **b** Biopsy histology (× 200)

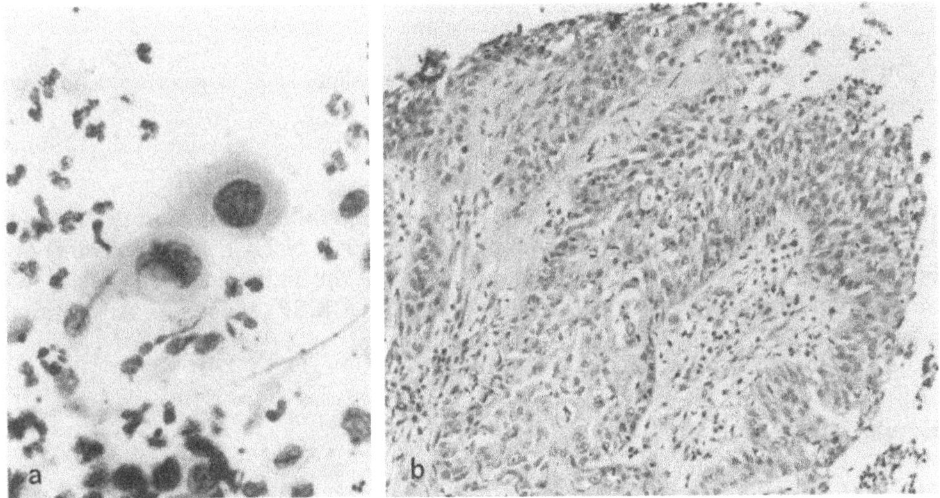

Fig. 8a, b. Invasive squamous cell carcinoma of beagle B6 after 30 weeks. Single cancer cells are observed. Histology shows submucosal invasion. **a** Brush cytology (× 400). **b** Biopsy histology (× 100)

Cytochemistry

Nuclear DNA measurements were performed in the different abnormal cell types observed during the carcinogenic process. Cells fulfilling the criteria described above

Pap.-stained slide
↓
Demounting in Xylol   10 h
↓

destaining of Papanicolaou
{
Xylol/abs. (1 : 1) → abs. → 95% al. → 70% al. → 50% al.   2 min each
↓
2 N HCl/70% al. (1 : 1)   15 min
↓
Aq. dest   several times
↓
}

Feulgen stain
{
Neutral Formalin (10% pH 6.9)   at least 10 h
↓
Aq. dest   several times
↓
5 N HCl (22° C) 1 h
↓
Aq. dest   several times
↓
Shiff reagent   2 h
↓
Aq. dest   (several times until the color of the solution has disappeared)
↓
Na₂S₂O₅-solution ×   3 times, 10 min each
↓   (newly made)
Tap water   5 min
↓
Aq. dest   1−2 min
↓
Mounting in D.P.X.
}

{
abs: absolute alcohol
al: alcohol
× 180 ml Aq. dest
   10 ml 1 N HCl
   110 ml 10% Na₂S₂O₅
}

Fig. 9. Procedure for destaining of Papanicolaou stained slides and Feulgen staining for cytophotometric DNA analysis

were selected from Papanicolaou stained smear preparations and were destained in
acidic alcohol, refixed in 10% formalin, hydrolyzed (5 N HCl, 22° C, 60 min) and
Feulgen stained (Fig. 9). Feulgen DNA content in individual cell nuclei was
determined by a microspectrophotometer (Olympus MMSP) at 546 nm. Adventitious
columnar cells were used as controls.

Results

Morphological Findings

First experimental group − six dogs (two beagles and four mongrels; Fig. 10).
In three dogs (two beagles and one mongrel) it was demonstrated cytologically and
histologically that invasive squamous cell carcinoma developed after the occurrence of
increasing degrees of atypia in immature and/or squamous metaplastic cells. In two of
the four mongrels, carcinoma in situ was diagnosed histologically.
In case 1 (beagle B5) mild atypical metaplasia was observed 1 week after the injection,
moderate atypia was seen after 3 weeks, severe atypia after 5 weeks, and carcinoma in

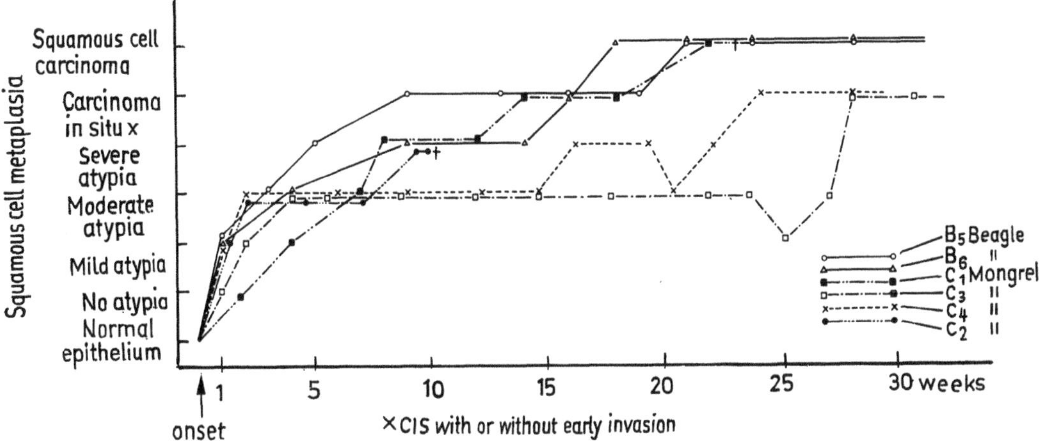

Fig. 10. The process of development of pulmonary squamous cell carcinoma in dogs according to time (weeks) and cellular atypia

situ after 9 weeks. Invasive squamous cell carcinoma was diagnosed cytologically and histologically 21 weeks after the commencement of the experiment.

In case 2 (beagle B6) mild atypical metaplasia appeared 1 week after the injection of 20-MC, moderate atypia after 4 weeks, severe atypia after 9 weeks, and carcinoma in situ after 16 weeks. Invasive squamous cell carcinoma was observed 18 weeks after the commencement of the experiment.

In case 3 (mongrel C1) regular metaplasia was observed after 1 week, mild atypia after 4 weeks, moderate atypia after 7 weeks, severe atypia after 8 weeks, carcinoma in situ after 15 weeks, and invasive squamous cell carcinoma after 22 weeks. Autopsy was performed 24 weeks after the commencement of the experiment. Autopsy showed early invasive squamous cell carcinoma, carcinoma in situ, various degrees of atypical metaplasia, and also basal cell hyperplasia in adjoining sites of the bronchus. Changes in the bronchial gland ducts were often more prominent than changes in the bronchial epithelium (Fig. 11).

In case 4 (mongrel C3) regular metaplasia was observed after 1 week, mild atypia after 2 weeks, moderate atypia after 4 weeks. After 25 weeks the atypia decreased temporarily. After 27 weeks moderate atypia was observed again and carcinoma in situ was demonstrated after 28 weeks. No invasive carcinoma has developed by the time of writing (after 80 weeks).

In case 5 (mongrel C4) regular metaplasia was observed after 1 week, mild atypia after 2 weeks, moderate atypia after 3 weeks, and severe atypia after 16 weeks. The severe atypia decreased to moderate after 20 weeks, but a progression to severe atypia occurred again after 22 weeks. Carcinoma in situ was observed after 24 weeks.

In case 6 (mongrel C2) mild atypical metaplasia was found after 1 week, moderate atypia after 2 weeks, and severe atypical metaplasia after 9 weeks. This case was autopsied but neither carcinoma in situ nor invasive squamous cell carcinoma was observed.

In this experiment with six dogs, basal cell hyperplasia with nuclear atypia was observed and was followed by atypical immature and/or squamous metaplasia after

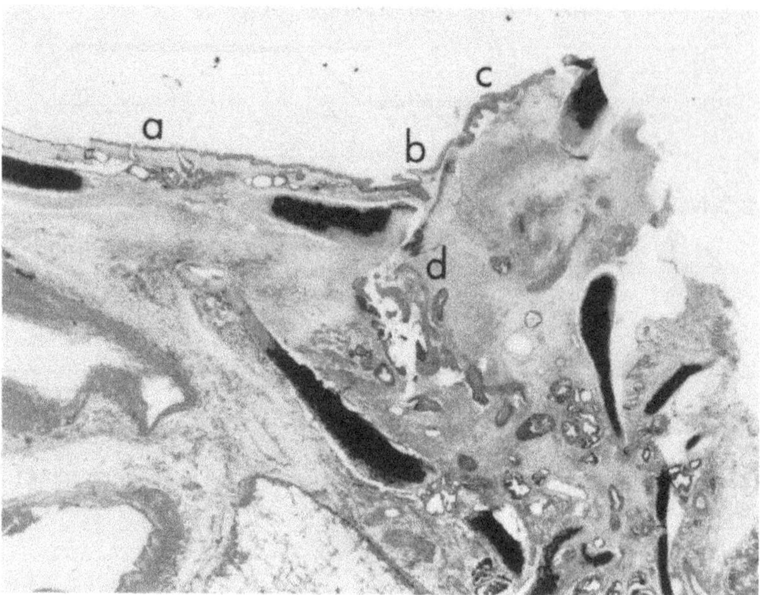

Fig. 11. Autopsy specimen of mongrel C1 after 24 weeks; *a,* normal epithelium; *b,* moderate atypical squamous metaplasia; *c,* carcinoma in situ; *d,* early invasive squamous cell carcinoma (× 10)

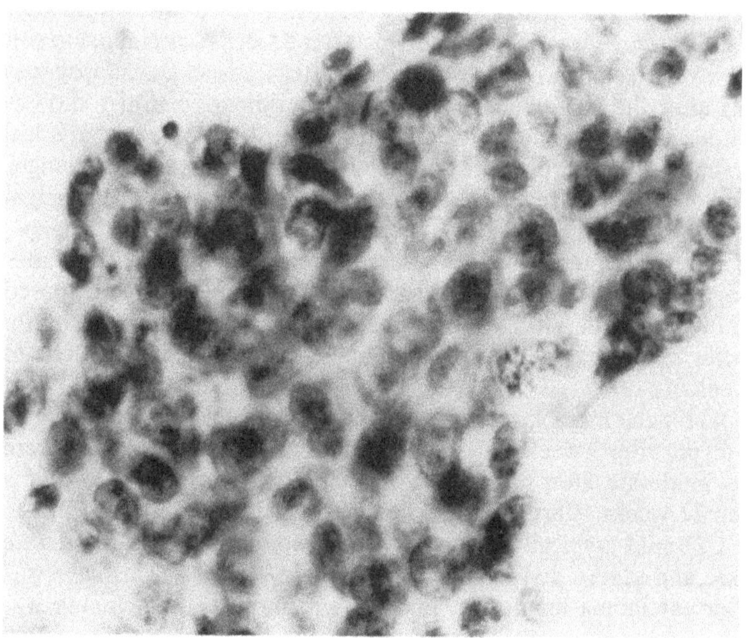

Fig. 12. Basal cell hyperplasia with nuclear atypia of beagle B9 after 1 day. Brush cytology (× 400)

Table 1. Bronchofiberscopic findings during the carcinogenetic process in dog

| | SQUAMOUS CELL METAPLASIA WITH | | | | | | | | | | | | | | | | | | | | | | | | | | | | CARCINOMA IN SITU* | | | | | | | SQUAMOUS CELL CARCINOMA | | | | | | |
	NO ATYPIA							MILD ATYPIA							MODERATE ATYPIA							SEVERE ATYPIA																				
	HYPEREMIA	PALENESS	DULLNESS	THICKENING	WIDENING OF SPUR	BLEEDING	IRREGULARITY	HYPEREMIA	PALENESS	DULLNESS	THICKENING	WIDENING OF SPUR	BLEEDING	IRREGULARITY	HYPEREMIA	PALENESS	DULLNESS	THICKENING	WIDENING OF SPUR	BLEEDING	IRREGULARITY	HYPEREMIA	PALENESS	DULLNESS	THICKENING	WIDENING OF SPUR	BLEEDING	IRREGULARITY	HYPEREMIA	PALENESS	DULLNESS	THICKENING	WIDENING OF SPUR	BLEEDING	IRREGULARITY	HYPEREMIA	PALENESS	DULLNESS	THICKENING	WIDENING OF SPUR	BLEEDING	IRREGULARITY
1 (B5)								−	+	−	−	−	−	−	−	+	−	+	−	−	+	−	+	−	+	−	−	+	−	+	+	+	+	−	#	+	−	−	#	+	+	#
2 (B6)								+	−	+	±	−	−	−	−	+	+	+	−	−	−	−	+	+	+	−	−	+	+	−	+	+	+	−	#	+	−	−	#	+	+	#
3 (C1)	−	+	−	−	−	−	−	−	+	+	−	−	−	−	−	+	+	+	−	−	±	−	+	+	+	−	−	±	−	−	+	+	−	−	+	+	−	−	#	−	+	#
4 (C3)	+	−	−	−	−	−	−	−	+	−	−	−	−	−	−	+	−	+	−	−	−								+	−	+	+	−	+	+							
5 (C4)	−	−	−	−	−	−	−	−	+	−	−	−	−	−	−	+	−	+	−	−	±	−	+	+	+	−	−	+	−	+	+	+	+	−	+							

± : SLIGHT # : STRONG
*CARCINOMA IN SITU WITH OR WITHOUT EARLY INVASION

weekly 20-MC injections. Nuclear atypia increased progressively during the carcinogenic process.

Second experimental group − two dogs (one beagle and one mongrel).
In this group, atypical basal cell hyperplasia was observed 1 day after 20-MC injections in both animals (Fig. 12). These alterations disappeared after 4 days and were successively replaced by immature and/or squamous metaplasia. The mongrel showed mild atypical metaplasia after 1 week and moderate atypia after 8 weeks. Finally a regression to mild atypia was demonstrated. In the beagle, regular metaplasia was observed after 1 week but reversed to normal after 4 weeks.

Third experimental group − two dogs (one beagle and one mongrel).
In this group atypical basal cell hyperplasia was found 1 day after the H_2O injection in both animals. Normal epithelium was observed after 4 days. Subsequently mild atypia was demonstrated up to 7 months, when this experiment was ended.

Fiberoptic Bronchoscopic Findings

Table 1 shows the fiberoptic bronchoscopic findings of the bronchial epithelial changes during the carcinogenic process. Almost no abnormal findings could be recognized in regular metaplasia, but paleness of the bronchial mucosa was seen in mild atypical metaplasia. In moderate atypical metaplasia (Fig. 13) paleness and thickening were observed. Paleness, dullness, thickening, and irregularity of the epithelium were observed in severe atypical metaplasia. In carcinoma in situ irregularity in addition to dullness and thickening was found (Fig. 14). Hyperemia, bleeding, severe thickening and irregularity was seen in invasive carcinoma (Fig. 15).

H. Kato et al.

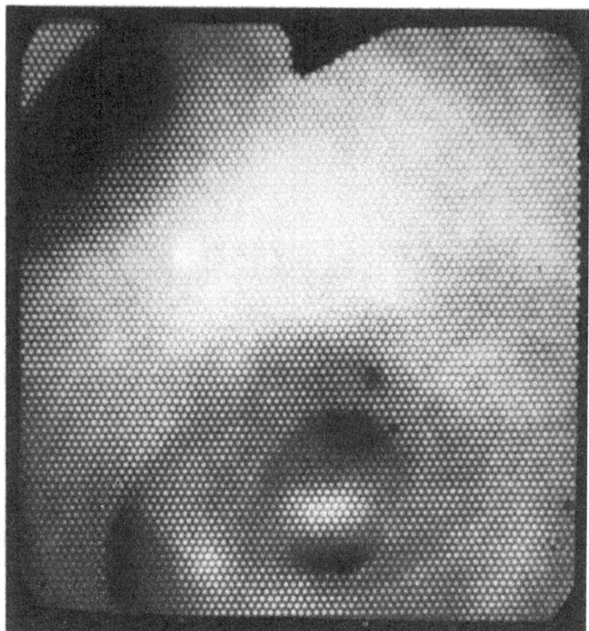

Fig. 13. Fiberoptic bronchoscopic findings of moderate atypical metaplasia of beagle B5 after 4 weeks. Paleness and thickening of the bronchial mucosa

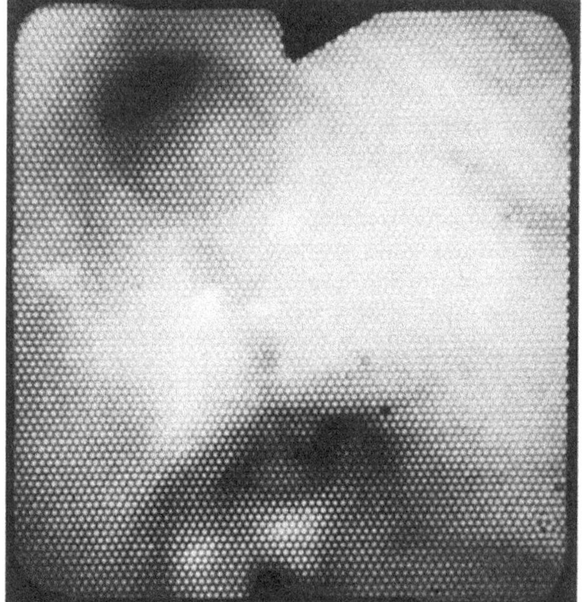

Fig. 14. Fiberoptic bronchoscopic findings of beagle B6 after 18 weeks show irregularity, thickening, and dullness of the mucosa. Diagnosis: carcinoma in situ

Cytophotometric DNA Analysis

The Feulgen nuclear DNA content was measured at various degrees of atypia in metaplastic cells, carcinoma in situ, and invasive carcinoma (Fig. 16).
In regular metaplastic cells, normal diploid DNA distribution patterns were observed.
Metaplastic cells with mild atypia showed DNA contents mainly between the diploid

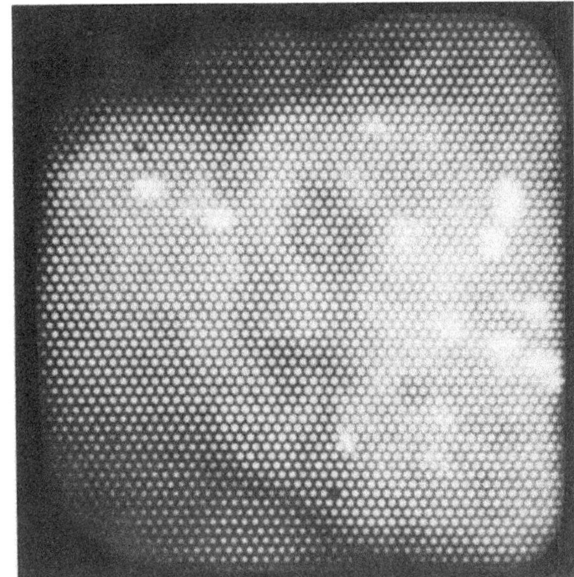

Fig. 15. Fiberoptic bronchoscopic findings of beagle B5 after 21 weeks show striking irregularity, thickening, and bleeding. Diagnosis: early invasive carcinoma

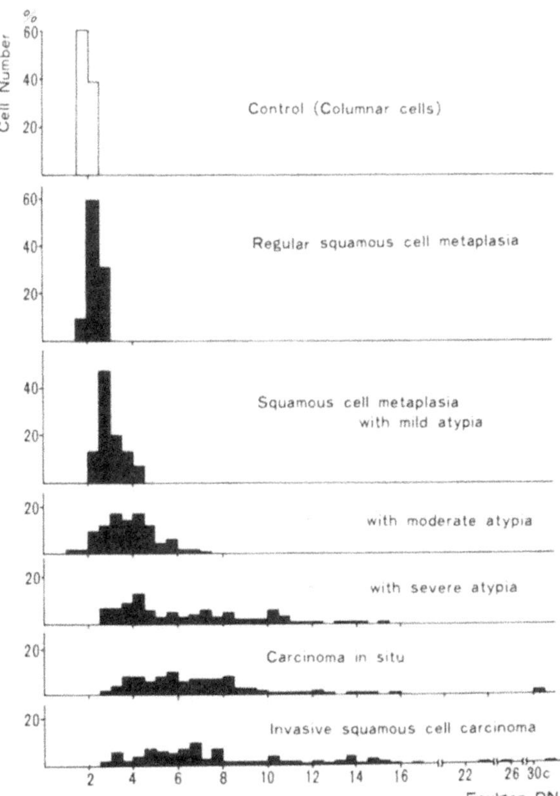

Fig. 16. Cytophotometric DNA analysis of metaplastic cells, cells indicating carcinoma in situ, and invasive carcinoma. Diploid cells decrease and heteroploid cells increase parallel with the progression of atypia in metaplastic cells

and triploid range. There was also a small number of cells in the tetraploid region. Feulgen DNA analysis of moderate atypical metaplasia showed the majority of the cells to be between the diploid and tetraploid regions with a small number of cells exceeding the 5C region. In severe atypical metaplasia cytophotometric analysis showed a heteroploid DNA distribution pattern without any cells in the diploid region. In carcinoma in situ and invasive squamous cell carcinoma the same heteroploid DNA distribution patterns were observed (Fig. 16).

Discussion

The cellular changes that occur during the pathogenesis of human pulmonary squamous cell carcinoma are to a large extent still unknown. Several investigators [1–3, 22, 23, 28] have reported that a high incidence of squamous metaplasia occurred in smokers and lung cancer patients and further studies indicated that squamous metaplasia, particularly metaplasia with cellular atypia, appeared to be a possible precursor to squamous cell carcinoma. Others [15, 32] have expressed criticism of the mechanism mentioned above partly because they did not observe squamous metaplasia or epithelial atypia in surrounding areas of carcinoma in situ or invasive carcinoma.

Several experiments [5–7, 18, 30, 31, 34] have been carried out to clarify this problem in small animals, but the value of these is limited as they do not permit monitoring of the carcinogenic process in the same animal. The present experiments were attempted, therefore, to induce central-type lung cancer in larger animals, i.e., dogs, to enable a chronological monitoring of the carcinogenic process at well defined sites in the bronchi. Such experiments using dogs were reported by Beattie and co-workers [4] among others [11, 12, 19, 25–27, 33], but the rates of cancer induction were low.

The carcinogen used in the present experiment was 20-MC. The authors have already reported a high rate of successful induction of peripheral-type lung cancer with this agent in rabbits and dogs. The dosage of 50 mg was selected because of the experience of previous experiments [18].

In the present experiments, three out of six dogs which received weekly injections of 20-MC developed carcinoma at 18, 21, and 22 weeks, respectively. Basal cell hyperplasia, with or without nuclear atypia, appeared shortly after injection of 20-MC, followed by immature and/or squamous metaplasia with increasing atypia during the carcinogenic process. Finally carcinoma in situ, in five dogs, and subsequently, in three dogs, early invasive squamous cell carcinoma developed (Fig. 17). It therefore seems that squamous metaplasia is a precursor of squamous cell carcinoma in this experimental model.

The fact that atypical metaplasia and basal cell hyperplasia adjacent to normal epithelium were observed surrounding the focus of carcinoma in autopsy material (mongrel C1) suggests that such cellular alterations may be precursor changes during the development of carcinoma.

The reason why changes in the bronchial gland ducts often were more pronounced than in the surface epithelium (Fig. 11) may be that the carcinogen was injected into the submucosa. The fact that atypical basal cell hyperplasia disappeared within a few days may be due to an unspecific, i.e., noncarcinogenic side effect of the carcinogen or admixed chemical substances, or to the physical stimulation caused by injection, and

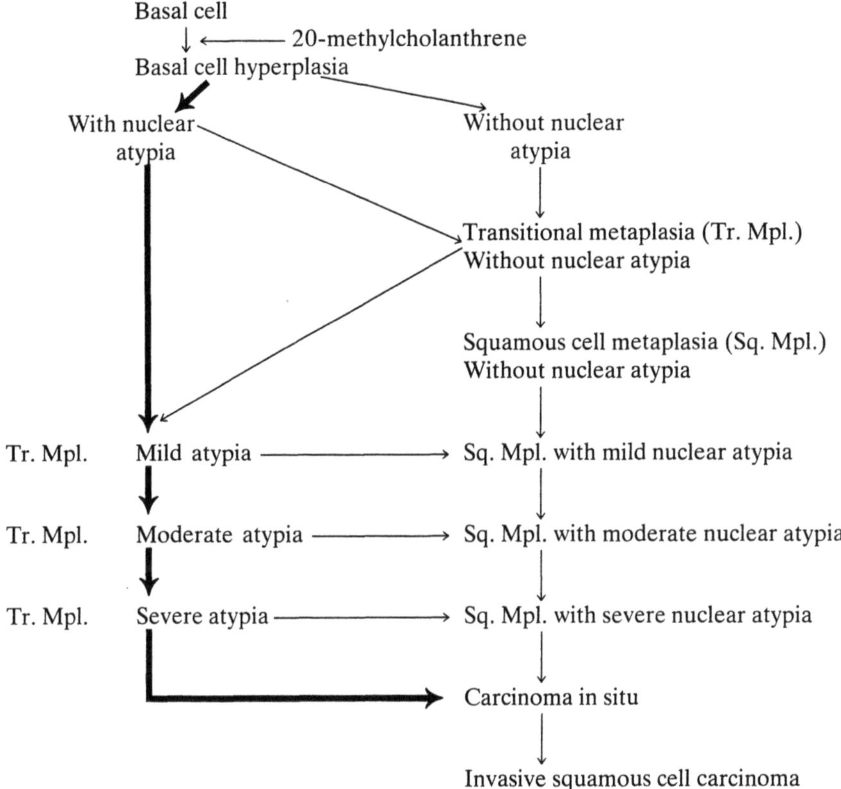

Fig. 17. Model of the carcinogenic process of experimental pulmonary squamous cell carcinoma in dogs

not due to its carcinogenic potential. The subsequent occurrence of regular or atypical metaplasia after 1 week may reflect specific carcinogenic changes due to the 20-MC remaining in the submucosa, but could also be explained by an unspecific growth stimulatory effect [13, 14]. No progressive changes were obtained by a single 20-MC injection. To obtain an increased atypia and induce carcinoma, repeated exposure to the carcinogen was found to be necessary.

In order to obtain additional and objective information about the nature of the carcinogenic process, the authors determined the amount of nuclear DNA at various degrees of nuclear atypia of metaplastic cells observed during the carcinogenic transformation, and of cells indicating carcinoma.

The DNA histograms of the pertinent cells indicate that the number of diploid cells decreases and the DNA distribution pattern becomes gradually more scattered as the degree of nuclear atypia increases. This means that the number of aneuploid cells which are frequently observed in cancer tends to increase gradually during the carcinogenic course.

Since morphologic alterations parallel changes in the DNA distribution patterns, it appears possible that atypical metaplasia may be transformed into carcinoma. This may indicate that cells with abnormal chromosomes already exist at the metaplastic stage of the carcinogenic process. The DNA distribution pattern in severe atypical metaplasia is approximately the same as in carcinoma in situ and invasive carcinoma. Severe atypical metaplasia, therefore, seems on cytophotometric evidence already to possess a malignant potential.

However, severe atypia regressed to a milder degree of atypia and carcinoma did not develop when the 20-MC injections were discontinued, as was shown in a previous study [8]. Thus, it is surmised that a defense mechanism against the development of carcinoma is still functioning at this stage. The development of carcinoma, therefore, is suggested to depend not only upon constant exposure to carcinogens, but also upon complicated host factors such as immunological potential, age, hormone, etc.

The fact that squamous metaplasia was seen in all dogs prior to the development of squamous cell carcinoma by no means shows that this is always the case in the development of human squamous cell carcinoma. It is possible that atypical squamous cell metaplasia is representative of unspecific effects and that squamous carcinoma might occur due to carcinogenic effects without the appearance of metaplasia.

This could lead to DNA abnormalities in some cells. Cells possessing autonomous proliferation abilities could then develop into cancer during the metaplastic process.

It is not clear how representative the present experimental lung cancer model is with respect to human carcinogenesis since the dosage of the carcinogen was high and administered at short intervals. Immature and/or squamous metaplasia, and particularly atypical metaplasia, is, however, considered to be a precursor of carcinoma according to the observations in the present experiment.

Acknowledgments. Supported in part by Grants-in-Aid for Cancer Research from the Ministry of Health and Welfare, Ministry of Education, the Japan Tobacco Monopoly Corporation, the Tokyo Medical College Cancer Center, and the Swedish Cancer Society.

References

1. Auer G, Kato H, Nasiell M, Roger V, Zetterberg A, Karlen L (1980) Cytophotometric DNA-analysis of atypical squamous metaplastic cells, carcinoma in situ, and bronchogenic carcinoma. In: Nieburgs HE (ed) Prevention and detection of cancer, vol 2/II. Marcel Dekker, New York Basel, pp 1465–1476
2. Auerbach O, Hammond EC (1970) Effects of cigarette smoking on dogs. Arch Environ Health 21: 754–768
3. Auerbach O, Gere JB, Forman JB et al. (1957) Changes in the bronchial epithelium in relation to smoking and cancer of the lung. N Engl J Med 254: 97–104
4. Beattie EJ, Staub EW, Correl N, Hass G (1961) Bronchogenic carcinoma produced experimentally in the dog. J Thorac Cardiovasc Surg 42: 615–622
5. Harris CC, Sporn MB, Kaufman DG, Smith JM, Jackson FE, Saffiotti U (1972) Histogenesis of squamous metaplasia in the hamster tracheal epithelium caused by Vitamin A deficiency or benzo(a)pyrene-ferric oxide. J Natl Cancer Inst. 48: 743–761
6. Harris CC, Kaufman DG, Sporn MB, Saffiotti U (1973a) Histogenesis of squamous metaplasia and squamous cell carcinoma of the respiratory epithelium in an animal model. Cancer Chemother Rep 4: 43–54
7. Harris CC, Kaufman DG, Sporn MB, Smith JM, Jackson F, Saffiotti U (1973b) Ultrastructural effect of N-methyl-N-nitrosourea on the tracheobronchial epithelium of the Syrian hamster. Int J Cancer 12: 259–269

8. Hayashi N, Hayata Y, Kawamura I, Kato H, Konaka C, Ono J (1974) Characteristics of 20-MC induced central type lung cancer in dogs. Proceedings of Jpn Cancer Assoc 39th Annual Meeting, 53
9. Hayata Y, Kato H, Chow M-C et al. (1977) Studies of the carcinogenetic process in experimental squamous cell carcinoma in canine lung. Jpn J Thorac Dis 15: 759−768
10. Kato H, Saito T, Ono J et al. (1980) Carcinogenetic process of central type squamous cell carcinoma in dogs and clinical application. Lung Cancer (Jpn) 20: 53−62
11. Kobayashi N, Kanisawa M, Okamoto T, Okita M, Katsuki H (1978a) Sequential cytologic study of the development of squamous cell carcinoma induced in subcutaneously implanted bronchial autograft of dogs. Acta Cytol (Baltimore) 22: 99−104
12. Kobayashi N, Okita T, Hanzawa S, Okamoto T, Katsuki H (1978b) A method for experimental injection of bronchogenic carcinoma in subcutaneously implanted bronchial autograft in dogs. J Thorac Cardiovasc Surg 75: 434−442
13. Konaka C, Auer G, Nasiell M et al. (to be published) Pathogenesis of squamous bronchial carcinoma in 20-methylcholanthrene-treated beagle dogs. Anal Quant Cytol
14. Konaka C, Auer G, Nasiell M, Hayata Y, Kato H, Caspersson T (to be published) Sequential cytomorphological and cytochemical changes during development of bronchial carcinoma in beagle dogs exposed to 20-methylcholanthrene. Cancer
15. Melamed MR, Zaman MB, Flehinger BJ, Martini N (1977) Radiologically occult in situ and incipient invasive epidermoid cancer. Am J Surg Pathol 1: 5−16
16. Müller K-M (1979a) Krebsvorstadien der Bronchialschleimhaut. Verh Dtsch Ges Pathol 63: 112−131
17. Müller K-M (1979b) Morphologie und Häufigkeit präinvasiver Neoplasien und früher Carcinome. In: Georgii A (Hrsg) Frühe Tumoren in Diagnostik und Therapie. Verh Dtsch Krebs-Ges, Bd 2. Fischer, Stuttgart New York
18. Nakajima H, Oho K, Chow M-C et al. (1975a) Experimental lung cancer induced in rabbits by intrabronchial application of 20-methylcholanthrene. Lung Cancer (Jpn) 15: 119−124
19. Nakajima H, Hayata Y, Hayashi N et al. (1975b) Experimental lung cancer produced in dogs by intrabronchial application of 20-methylcholanthrene-technique and characteristics of induced tumors. Lung Cancer (Jpn) 15: 53−59
20. Nasiell M (1963) The general appearance of the bronchial epithelium in bronchial carcinoma: a histopathological study with some cytological viewpoints. Acta Cytol (Baltimore) 7: 97−106
21. Nasiell M (1966) Metaplasia and atypical metaplasia in the bronchial epithelium. A histopathologic and cytopathologic study. Acta Cytol (Baltimore) 10: 421−427
22. Nasiell M (1968) Comparative histological and sputumcytological studies of the bronchial epithelium in inflammatory and neoplastic lung disease. Acta Pathol Microbiol Scand 72: 501−518
23. Nasiell M, Kato H, Auer G, Zetterberg A, Roger V, Karlen L (1978) Cytomorphological grading and Feulgen DNA-analysis of metaplastic and neoplastic bronchial cells. Cancer 41: 1511−1521
24. Nettesheim P, Griesemer RA, Martin DH, Caton JE Jr (1977) Induction of preneoplastic and neoplastic lesions in grafted rat tracheas continuously exposed to benzo(a)pyrene. Cancer Res 37: 1272−1278
25. Okita M, Cohen AH, Benfield JR (1974) Localized submucosal bronchial injections of carcinogens in dogs. In: Karbe E, Park JF (eds) Experimental lung cancer. Springer, Berlin Heidelberg New York, pp 102−115
26. Rigdon RH, Crossen G (1963) Pulmonary lesions in dogs from methylcholanthrene. Arch Pathol 75: 323−331
27. Rockey EE, Kuschner M, Kosak AL, Mayer E (1958) The effect of tobacco tar on the bronchial mucosa of dogs. Cancer 11: 466−472
28. Saccomanno G, Archer VC, Auerbach O, Saunders RP, Brennan LM (1974) Development of carcinoma of the lung as reflected in exfoliated cells. Cancer 33: 256−270

29. Saccomanno G (1978) Diagnostic pulmonary cytology. Am Soc Clin Pathol, Chicago
30. Saffiotti U, Montesano R, Sellakumar AR, Borg SA (1967) Experimental cancer of the lung. Inhibition by vitamin A of the induction of tracheobronchial squamous metaplasia and squamous cell tumors. Cancer 20: 857–864
31. Schreiber H, Saccomanno G, Martin DH, Brennan L (1974) Sequential cytological changes during development of respiratory tract tumors induced in hamsters by benzo(a)pyrene ferric oxide. Cancer Res 34: 689–698
32. Shimosato Y (1980) Growth characteristics, prognosis and functions of lung cancer in relation to its morphology. Lung Cancer (Jpn) 20: 3–20
33. Staub EW, Eisenstein R, Hass G, Beattie EJ (1972) Bronchogenic carcinoma produced experimentally in the normal dog. J Thorac Cardiovasc Surg 49: 364–372
34. Stenbäck F, Sellakumar A (1974) Squamous metaplasia and respiratory tumor induced by intratracheal instillation of 7,12-dimethyl-(a)-anthracene in Syrian golden hamsters. Eur J Cancer 10: 483–486

Bronchoscopic Localization
of Radiologically Occult Cancer*

B. Marsh, J. Frost, and Y. Erozan

The Johns Hopkins Hospital, Baltimore, MD, USA

Bronchoscopy has played a long and important role in the study of patients with clinical bronchogenic carcinoma. It is well known, however, that some bronchial carcinomas shed malignant cells into the sputum for periods of many months before becoming detectable by bronchoscopy or chest X-ray [1]. Prior to the advent of the fiberoptic bronchoscope, differential cytology was too unreliable to allow definitive therapy in such patients until biopsy confirmation could be made.
The Johns Hopkins Lung Project is a lung cancer screening study of male cigarette smokers over 45 years of age. Those individuals whose sputum cytology contains malignant cells and whose chest X-ray is unrevealing are referred for bronchoscopic localization studies.
It is the purpose of this paper to outline the localization methods developed and to focus on bronchoscopic results obtained in our study of 55 men harboring radiographically occult tumors. This group includes both screens of the project (45 cases), and referrals to us from other sources (10 cases).

Method

Patients harboring malignant cells in their sputum are given a thorough medical evaluation with chest radiographs and are referred to our otolaryngologist for a detailed examination of the upper respiratory tract. The nasopharynx and larynx are carefully inspected with telescopes and mirrors for areas of irregularity, induration, tenderness, and friability. When this study has been completed bronchoscopy is performed. While local anesthesia will suffice in some cases, if no lesion is discovered a rather detailed study is required and general anesthesia needed. This provides (1) a quiet tracheobronchial tree for "uncontaminated" brush specimens; (2) optimal conditions for an unhurried examination of each segment and retrieval of as many specimens as necessary; and (3) opportunity to perform a direct laryngoscopy and obtain specimens from the upper respiratory tract as well. We use a 9-mm endotracheal tube through which localized bronchoscopic specimens of optimal quality and reliability can be obtained.

---

* This work was supported in part by the National Cancer Institute Contract NIH 69-2172

A careful search of all bronchi is conducted with special attention to segmental spurs where the earliest changes of neoplasia are frequently observed. In most adults one can reach the subsegmental level, which is usually sufficient to find squamous carcinomas whose exfoliated cells reach the sputum.

While many of these lesions can be recognized by the well trained bronchoscopist, they are frequently inconspicuous and sometimes completely invisible. In such cases we require a dependable method for obtaining "uncontaminated" cells from each bronchus, and the following procedure has proven both effective and reliable. Following completion of the visual search, we flush the bronchoscopic channel with a balanced salt solution and insert a clean brush into the channel, where it remains protected until positioned at the bronchus to be studied. Here the brush is passed from the lumen of the bronchoscope into all accessible segments of the lobe to be studied and then pulled back just to the tip of the bronchoscope. The two are then removed and the specimen dislodged from the brush before it is withdrawn from the instrument. The channel is again flushed to remove any cells and a new brush inserted. Each lobe is then sampled in this fashion and separate specimens also obtained from the superior segments and lingula as well. Microbiopsies are then obtained from any suspicious areas including localized areas of bleeding from the brushing procedure, and may also be obtained from representative sites at the segmental level of each lobe.

If a tumor is identified, we anticipate where the bronchus might be severed during a subsequent resection. Not infrequently very small lesions of the lobar and segmental bronchi may be associated with an unsuspected extension of carcinoma in situ into a more proximal bronchus [2]. A biopsy of the lobar spur may detect this condition and suggest the need for more than a simple lobectomy in order to obtain a tumor-free margin.

If no suspicion of tumor is found in the lung, a direct laryngoscopy is performed, and cytologic smears are obtained from the nasopharynx as well.

Results

In a group of 55 patients, 39 were found to harbor tumors of the bronchi. Seven of these tumors were multifocal, occurring in at least two areas widely separated from each other. Except for one patient with adenocarcinoma, all were squamous carcinomas. The majority (33/39) of these tumors appeared to originate in the segmental bronchi, and most were near a bifurcation from the lobar bronchi. We found a few surprisingly large tumors involving major bronchi, while others were no more than a patch of carcinoma in situ hidden in a small segmental bronchus. In the least extensive lesions we observed only slight capillary irregularity or localized mucosal friability. Thickening of a segmental spur or narrowing of a bronchial orifice also suggest early tumor. The brush specimens were remarkably accurate in identifying the involved bronchus or bronchi whether or not a lesion could be seen. In no case did brush material provide a false positive localization. Most of the larger tumors were found in our prevalence cases, while tumors discovered after several years of periodic surveillance by sputum cytology were nearly all in situ with little or no invasion demonstrated in the resected specimens.

There were 11 of the 55 whose source of malignant cells was discovered in the upper respiratory tract, including the larynx, pharynx, and nasopharynx. Three of these required direct laryngoscopy for confirmation. Most were early-stage tumors with an optimistic prognosis.

In two subjects whose sputum cytology showed malignant cells, the malignancy could not be localized. In neither of these were we able to obtain any malignant cells by endoscopic procedures performed. In both the sputum reverted to moderately atypical cells and remained in that category until this report 3 years later. Within the past week, one of these is again showing malignant cells in the sputum and a repeat localization attempt is being scheduled. The final result in these two patients has yet to be determined.

Three subjects are considered localization failures:

Case 1. A 69-year-old man was referred to us to discover the source of squamous carcinoma cells found in the sputum. At bronchoscopy no lesion was found and no malignant cells retrieved from multiple brushings. He also had adenocarcinoma of the prostate and was lost to follow-up.

Case 2. A 51-year-old man had a right lower lobe previously removed for adenocarcinoma. When his sputum subsequently revealed adenocarcinoma cells without radiographic changes, we attempted bronchoscopic localization. No endo-bronchial lesions were found, but the brush specimens from the right upper lobe showed "marked atypia". A repeat localization attempt several months later revealed adenocarcinoma cells from the right upper lobe, but his admission chest X-ray already demonstrated a small right upper lobe lesion.

Case 3. A 60-year-old man was referred for our aid in localizing the source of squamous carcinoma cells found in the sputum. Repeated bronchoscopic brushings and studies of the upper respiratory tract failed to obtain malignant cells. He soon revealed a 5-cm mass in the superior segment, left lower lobe (LB-6a). This area is notoriously difficult to reach with our instruments, and we clearly had failed to brush the involved subsegment. When this lesion was seen on X-ray, we were successful in obtaining a diagnostic biopsy at bronchoscopy. At autopsy, microscopic studies revealed small undifferentiated carcinoma with areas of large cell undifferentiated carcinoma, squamous cell carcinoma, and adenocarcinoma.

Summary

The fiberoptic bronchoscope has greatly extended our capabilities for the diagnosis of lung cancer, especially in the early segmental lesions. Most of those that are manifest only by sputum cytology can now be localized by a technique sufficiently reliable to allow definitive therapy.

References

1. Pearson FW, Thompson DW, Delarue NC (1967) Experience with the cytologic detection, localization and treatment of radiologically undemonstrated bronchial carcinoma. J Thorac Cardiovasc Surg 54: 371–382
2. Straus MJ (1977) Lung cancer clinical diagnosis and treatment. Grune and Stratton, New York San Francisco London, p 111

Hematoporphyrin Derivative as a Tumor Marker in the Detection and Localization of Pulmonary Malignancy

E. G. King, D. Doiron, G. Man, A. E. Profio, and G. Huth*

University of Alberta, Edmonton, Alberta, Canada

Although a number of compounds, including eosin [14, 35], fluorescein [7, 26], tetracyclines [32, 37], and acridine orange [36], are known to induce fluorescence in tumors, the porphyrins have received greatest attention. Of this latter group, hematoporphyrin and its derivatives seem to be the most effective in inducing fluorescence [1, 2, 11, 38] and therefore have been considered the most likely to prove useful in the detection and localization of lung tumors. Equally of interest are the photodynamic properties of porphyrins which, when concentrated and localized within tumor tissue, render the malignancy susceptible to phototherapy [8].

Historical Perspective

In 1942 Policard noted that human tumors demonstrated red fluorescence when illuminated with ultraviolet light, whereas normal tissue did not [29]: this observed fluorescence was linked to a porphyrin compound. In 1942, Auler and Banzer [1] and Figge [10] showed that administration of some natural porphyrins could produce bright red fluorescence in animal tumors; Figge also noted that hematoporphyrin was more successful in localizing a variety of induced mouse tumors (fibrosarcoma and mammary carcinoma) than were coproporphyrin, protoporphyrin, or mesoporphyrin. Hematoporphyrin was observed to localize in embryonic tissue, lymph nodes, and traumatized tissue [11].

In the 1950s a number of studies employed hematoporphyrin to detect a variety of tumors [25, 27, 28, 33]. These effects met with variable success and the ideal dosage, material, and route of administration remained uncertain. Hematoporphyrin was also tried as a tumor sensitizer, but for radiation rather than phototherapy [24]. This too met with only low-key success, although tumors were again noted to fluoresce and the tumor response time and clinical course may have been marginally improved.

In 1961, Lipson [20] introduced a derivative of hematoporphyrin prepared by an acetic acid-sulfuric acid treatment of hematoporphyrin hydrochloride. The compound was

---

* The authors would like to thank Mrs. Darlene Odynski, Mrs. Ruby Miller, Drs. Jean leRiche and Roger Amy, and Mrs. Margaret Napier for their participation in the study reported in the review

termed hematoporphyrin derivative (Hpd) and was found to be a superior tumor localizer when compared to the parent hematoporphyrin. Lipson's group reported the use of Hpd for the detection of esophageal and tracheobronchial tumors in 15 patients. The major limitation in this and later studies was in the provision of adequate activating light by way of a quartz rod through the endoscope. There were no false positive results but four patients with negative fluorescence were shown to have malignancy. This study was expanded [21] in 1964 to include a further 35 patients known to have or suspected of having a neoplasm of the esophagus or tracheo-bronchial tree. For the total of 50 patients, positive fluorescence detection of malignant lesions was achieved in 32. Negative fluorescence was recorded in eight benign lesions and in one patient with coughed sputum cytologically positive for malignancy. Eight false negatives occurred, most thought to be due to insufficient activating violet light reaching the lesion. Hpd was also used by Lipson and his group for the detection and localization of cervical cancer, positive fluorescence being recorded in 29 of 31 patients with confirmed malignant disease [22]. False positive fluorescence occurred in 10 other patients in this series, biopsy demonstrating marked atypism in seven of these.

In 1967, Lipson et al. [23] reviewed their results in a cumulative total of 121 patients given Hpd for the detection of a variety of cancers, including esophagus, airways, rectum, peritoneal cavity, breast, tonsil, and parotid. For 113 accessible lesions, they reported 95% positive fluorescence detection for benign lesions. All positive benign cases were for lesions of the cervix or vagina, of which nine showed atypism and one showed chronic inflammation.

In 1968, Gray et al. reported the use of Hpd in 44 patients suspected of having a neoplastic lesion of the cervix [12]. Eighteen of the 23 positively diagnosed cancers showed positive fluorescence. The five false negatives occurring in this series were blamed on an inferior batch of Hpd and procedural errors. In the remaining 21 cases, nine of 11 with cellular dysplasia showed positive fluorescence while two of 10 patients with cervicitis fluoresced.

In the same year Gregorie et al. [13] published a large human study employing Hpd in cancer localization. The study included 266 patients with a wide variety of tumor types and locations. Of the 173 patients with malignancy, 132 (76%) demonstrated positive tumor fluorescence. Of the 41 false negative cases, 18 were thought to be due to inadequate illumination, insufficient drug administration, and bleeding. In 21 cases, endoscopic scanning was used for lesions of the esophagus, bronchus, and larynx. Sixteen of these 21 showed positive fluorescence. For the benign lesions studied, only 26% showed positive fluorescence and in most this was faint.

In 1971, Leonard and Beck reported a study of 40 patients with suspected cancerous lesions of the mouth, pharynx, hypopharynx, and larynx employing Hpd [19]. Positive fluorescence was noted in all 29 malignant lesions. Fluorescence was absent in three benign lesions and in four cases of inflammation. The two false positives were in prominent lymphoid tissue at the base of the tongue. Faint fluorescence at the base of the tongue had also been noted by previous workers [20].

Kyriazis, Balin, and Lipson reported a study in 1973 of the correlation between Hpd fluorescence and colposcopic, cytologic, and histopathologic findings in 20 patients with cervical atypism [18]. Positive fluorescence was noted in 15 of 16 cases which ranged in atypicality from moderate squamous metaplasia to carcinoma in situ. Also noted was positive fluorescence in one of three cases of chronic cervicitis and in one case with normal cytologic findings.

Kelly and Small used Hpd as a tumor marker in 11 patients suspected of having bladder cancer in 1976 [15]. Only faint fluorescence could be appreciated cystoscopically owing to inadequate illumination. Bladder examination after resection showed intense fluorescence in abnormal areas ranging from hyperplastic mucosa, through carcinoma in situ, to invasive carcinoma.

In the 1970s two groups have actively continued to use Hpd in the detection and localization of pulmonary tumors, with special attention directed toward occult malignancy of the airways. The Mayo Clinic group recognized early in the decade that standard glass fiberoptics did not efficiently transmit light in the violet range. In view of the fact that Hpd is optimally excited by the violet end of the light spectrum, they had Olympus Corporation develop a special bronchoscope with enhanced blue-violet range transmission capability [3, 34]. Despite this advance, light transmission and faint fluorescence imaging remained a major problem. More recently, the Mayo Group have developed an auditory nonimaging method for detecting Hpd airway tumor fluorescence during fiberoptic bronchoscopy [4, 5, 17]. This method is useful in directing white light examination of the airways, but does not allow actual visualization of the fluorescing area as a guide to biopsy.

Our group is an amalgam of workers at the Universities of Southern California and Alberta, and the Roswell Park Memorial Institute [6, 16, 30, 31]. It was clear from the earlier work cited in this review that one of the major problems preventing more useful clinical application of Hpd as a tumor marker was the detection of low levels of fluorescence from malignant cells. Attention was directed toward optimization of monochromatic light production and, in addition, fluorescence visualization was enhanced through use of an image intensifier system. The most recent advance in illumination came with the application of a krypton laser as a nearly monochromatic light source together with a single fused quartz fiberoptic light conductor that could be passed through the side channel of a standard Olympus BFB3 bronchoscope. Results of employing this technologically sophisticated approach to the detection and localization of cancer of the airways in 15 patients are briefly outlined below.

Illumination and Imaging System

Initial studies on 13 patients were performed with a mercury vapor lamp as a violet light source. This was a 200-W, high pressure, short-arc lamp with appropriate collimating and condensing lenses and a series of filters that selectively passed violet exciting light while rejecting the red portion of the spectrum. The laser system used for the last two patients in this study consisted of a krypton ion laser, violet filter, converging lens, and fused quartz fiber. The laser was a Spectra-Physics Model 164-11/265 which has special mirrors and a high field magnet for lasing in the violet. Output was in the order of 240 mW in three lines, 406.7 nm (36%), 413.1 nm (60%), and 415.4 nm (4%). The lens focuses the beam onto the 400-μm core of the fused quartz fiber. Overall diameter of the clad fiber is only 850 μm, making it small enough to be easily passed through the working side channel of a standard fiberoptic bronchoscope. Although the side channel can continue to be used for suctioning, brush and bite biopsy could only be carried out after first removing the fiber. A more recent dual channel fiberoptic bronchoscope obviates this problem. Approximately 10 mW are delivered to the illuminated surface.

The imaging portion of the system includes the standard objective lens and coherent fiberoptic bundle of the flexible fiberoptic bronchoscope (Olympus BFB3). The image is then magnified ($\times 2$) and focused on the fiberoptic faceplate of the intensifier, after passing through a red barrier filter to reject reflected violet and other nonred background. Either a broad band (600–700 nm) or narrow band (690–700 nm) nonfluorescent interference filter could be inserted by moving a slide. For general viewing and exploration of the airway, the broad band filter was used: if fluorescence was seen, the validity of the observation could be checked by sliding the narrow band filter with its superior signal-to-background ratio into place. The image intensifier is a three-stage, electrostatic focus type (Varo 8858) originally designed as a starlight illumination "sniperscope". The red response photocathode converts light energy to electrons which are then accelerated and focused onto a green phosphor screen, thereby converting a faint red image into a bright green one, the gain being in the order of 30,000.

Hematoporphyrin Derivative

Hpd was obtained from two sources: the first five patients received material prepared by Dr. J. C. Kennedy of Queen's University, Kingston, Ontario. The latter 10 patients received Hpd made by Dr. T. J. Dougherty of Roswell Park Memorial Institute, Buffalo, New York. This material was reconstituted, diluted, pyrogen-tested, and frozen for use; 1.5–2.5 mg/kg were administered to patients over a half hour into a freely running intravenous line. Hpd injection was timed to occur 48–72 h prior to bronchoscopy.

Patients and Procedure

Patients entering the pilot study were those in whom abnormal coughed sputum cytology had been documented or in whom there was reason to suspect the possible or probable presence of an endobronchial malignancy. Informed consent was obtained and patients were instructed to remain out of the sun and avoid bright incandescent light exposure for 3 weeks after Hpd injection.

All subjects initially underwent standard white light examination of their airways, following which the light source was switched from the Olympus CLS to either the mercury arc or laser system and the image intensifier applied to the eyepiece of the bronchoscope.

Results

Four of the 15 patients developed photosensitivity reactions ranging in severity from mild facial erythema (one patient) to severe blister formation (one patient). Another patient had a small amount of infused Hpd and intravenous fluid extravasate and this produced a red, swollen, painful area accompanied by fever. Table 1 summarizes the experimental record for the 15 patients. "Biopsy" refers to the results of brush or bite biopsy from an area of mucosa or tumor that either fluoresced or was abnormal on white light bronchoscopy. Generally, fluorescence was detected whenever tumor was

E. G. King et al.

Table 1. Summary of results

Pat. no.	Chest X-ray	Hpd (mg/kg)	WLB	FB	Biopsy
1	Mass RUL	1.5	+	+	Benign atypia
2	Clear	1.5	−	−	Benign atypia
3	Mass LUL	1.7	+	+	Small cell anaplastic
4	Mass LUL	1.7	+	+	Squamous cell ca
5	L hilar mass	1.4	+	+	Large cell anaplastic
6	LLL infiltrate	1.5	−	−	Inflammation
7	Clear	1.5	+	+	Squamous cell ca
8	Clear	2.5	+	+	Squamous cell ca
9	L hilar mass	2.5	−	−	Squamous cell ca
10	Clear	2.5	−	−	Benign atypia
11	Clear	2.5	+	+	Benign atypia
12	Atelectasis LLL	2.5	+	+	Small cell anaplastic
13	L pleural effusion	2.5	+	+	Adenocarcinoma
14	Clear	2.5	+	+	Squamous cell ca; dysplastic cells in sputum
15	Clear for ca	2.0	+	+	Squamous cell ca; pos. coughed sputum

WLB, White light bronchoscopy
FB, Fluorescence bronchoscopy

found to be present. Of the 10 patients shown to have malignancy of their airways, nine demonstrated tumor fluorescence. One patient in particular illustrated the sensitivity of the technique in that it was possible to demonstrate a small region of mucosal fluorescence within the posteroapical segment of the right upper lobe which on biopsy proved to be a squamous cell carcinoma. Serial section of the resection specimen showed that only minimally invasive squamous cell carcinoma (maximum penetration 1−1.5 mm) and carcinoma in situ were present, the region precisely conforming to the area of fluorescence noted in bronchoscopy.

Discussion

It is clearly apparent that Hpd is a potentially useful tumor marker for the production of fluorescence in the detection and localization of a variety of cancers, including malignancy of the airways (see also the paper by Dr. O. Balchum in this Symposium). This approach may be of particular value in the identification and localization of occult lung tumors in patients with coughed sputum cytology positive for malignancy but with negative chest X-ray and negative conventional fiberoptic bronchoscopic examination. What is equally exciting however is that the same basic principles used in detection and localization of tumors with Hpd may also be used for phototherapy. Dr. T. Dougherty at Roswell Park, Dr. J. Kennedy at Queen's University, Kingston, and Dr. I. Forbes in Adelaide have successfully produced tumor necrosis with phototherapy in Hpd injected patients [9], and Dr. Y. Hayata's group at the Tokyo Medical College have successfully used phototherapy in the management of malignancy of the airways (personal communication). Thus, the potential exists for Hpd as a fluorescence inducer to be useful in detection and localization, and as a photosensitizer in therapy. Much remains to be learned about the active principle and further purification of Hpd, its kinetics, the basis for tumor localization, and the optimal time for viewing and phototherapy. Further development in illumination, detection and imaging systems is essential. The last word has yet to be written on this intriguing compound: it will be interesting to follow its development as an example of Ehrlich's "magic-bullets" in diagnosis and therapy over the next few years.

References

1. Auler H, Banzer G (1942) Untersuchungen über die Rolle der Porphine bei geschwulstkranken Menschen und Tieren. Abh Krebsforsch 53: 65−68
2. Bases R, Brodie SS, Rubenfelds S (1958) Attempts at tumour localization using Cu-64-labelled copper porphyrins. Cancer 11: 259−263
3. Carpenter RJ, Neel HB, Ryan RJ, Sanderson DR (1977) Tumour fluorescence in vivo and in vitro with hematoporphyrin derivative. Ann Otol Rhinol Laryngol 86: 661−667
4. Cortese DA, Kinsey JH, Woolner LB, Payne WS, Sanderson DR, Fontana RS (1979) Clinical application of a new endoscopic technique for detection of in-situ bronchial carcinoma. Mayo Clin Proc 54: 635−642
5. Cortese DA, Kinsey JH (1981) Hematoporphyrin derivative fluorescence for lung cancer localization. Semin Resp Med 3/1: 37−44
6. Doiron DR, Profio AE, Vincent RG, Dougherty TJ (1979) Fluorescence bronchoscopy for detection of lung cancer. Chest 76: 27−32
7. Dougherty TJ (1974) Activated dyes as antitumour agents. J Natl Cancer Inst 52: 1333−1336
8. Dougherty TJ, Kaufman JE, Goldfarb A et al. (1978) Photoradiation therapy for the treatment of malignant tumours. Cancer Res 38: 2628−2635
9. Dougherty TJ, Weishaupt KR, Boyle DG (to be published) Photoradiation therapy of malignant tumours. Princ Pract Oncol
10. Figge RH (1942) Near ultraviolet light rays and fluorescence phenomena as aids to discovery and diagnosis in medicine. Univ Md Med Bull 26: 165
11. Figge RH, Weiland GS, Manganiello LOJ (1948) Cancer detection and therapy. Affinity of neoplastic, embryonic and traumatized tissues for porphyrins and metallophorphyrins. Proc Soc Exp Biol Med 68: 640−641
12. Gray MJ, Lipson RL, Mack JVS, Parker L, Rombyn D (1967) Use of hematoporphyrin derivative in detection and management of cervical cancer. Am J Obstet Gynecol 9: 766−771
13. Gregorie HB, Horger EO, Ward JL et al. (1968) Hematoporphyrin derivative fluorescence in malignant neoplasms. Ann Surg 167: 820−828
14. Jesionek A, von Tappeiner H (1904, 1905) Zur Behandlung der Hautcarcinome mit fluorescierenden Stoffen. Dtsch Arch Klin Med 82: 233−239
15. Kelly JF, Snell MB (1976) Hematoporphyrin derivative: a possible aid in the diagnosis and therapy of carcinoma of the bladder. J Urol 115: 150−151
16. King EG, Man G, LeRiche J et al. (to be published) Fluorescence bronchoscopy in the localization of bronchogenic carcinoma. Cancer
17. Kinsey JH, Cortese DA, Sanderson DR (1978) Detection of hematoporphyrin fluorescence during fiberoptic bronchoscopy to localize early bronchogenic carcinoma. Mayo Clin Proc 53: 594−600
18. Kyriazis GA, Balin H, Lipson RL (1973) Hematoporphyrin derivative-fluorescence test. Colposcopy and colpophotography in the diagnosis of atypical metaplasia, dysplasia and carcinoma in-situ of the cervix uteri. Am J Obstet Gynecol 117: 375−380

19. Leonard JR, Beck WL (1971) Hematoporphyrin fluorescence: an aid in diagnosis of malignant neoplasms. Laryngoscope 81: 365–377
20. Lipson RL, Baldes BJ, Olsen AM (1961) A new aid for endoscopic detection of malignant disease. J Thorac Cardiovasc Surg 42: 623–629
21. Lipson RL, Baldes BJ, Olsen AM (1964a) A further evaluation of the use of hematoporphyrin derivative as a new aid for the endoscopic detection of malignant disease. Dis Chest 46: 676–679
22. Lipson RL, Pratt JH, Balder BJ, Docherty MB (1964b) Hematoporphyrin derivative for detection of cervical cancer. Obstet Gynecol 24: 78–84
23. Lipson RL, Baldes BJ, Gray MJ (1967) Hematoporphyrin derivative for detection and management of cancer. Cancer 26: 2255–2257
24. Mack HP, Diehl WK, Peck GC, Figge H (1957) Hematoporphyrin and radiation treatment of carcinoma of the cervix. Cancer 10: 529–539
25. Mellors RC, Glassman A, Papanicolaou GN (1952) A microfluorometric scanning method for the detection of cancer cells in smears of exfoliated cells. Cancer 5: 458–468
26. Moore GB (1953) Diagnosis and localization of brain tumours; a clinical and experimental study employing fluorescent and radioactive tracer methods. Ch. Thomas, Springfield
27. Peck GC, Mack HP, Figge FH (1953) Cancer detection and therapy III. Affinity of lymphatic tissues for hematoporphyrin. Bull Sch Med Univ Md 38: 124–127
28. Peck GC, Mack HP, Holbrook WA, Figge FH (1955) Use of hematoporphyrin fluorescence in biliary and cancer surgery. Ann Surg 21: 181–188
29. Policard A (1924) Etudes sur les aspects offerts par des tumeurs experimentales examinées à la lumière de Woods. C R Soc Biol (Paris) 91: 1423–1424
30. Profio AE, Doiron DR (1977) A feasibility study of the use of fluorescence bronchoscopy for localization of small lung tumours. Phys Med Biol 22: 949–957
31. Profio AE, Doiron DR, King EG (1979) Laser fluorescence bronchoscope for localization of occult lung tumours. Med Phys 6: 523–525
32. Rall DD, Loo TL, Lane M, Kelly MG (1957) Appearance and persistence of fluorescent material in tumour tissue after tetracycline administration. J Natl Cancer Inst 19: 79–86
33. Rassmussen-Taxdal DS, Ward GR, Figge FH (1958) Fluorescence of human lymphatic and cancer tissue following high doses of intravenous hematoporphyrin. Cancer 8: 78–81
34. Sanderson DR, Fontanta RS, Lipson RL, Baldes BJ (1972) Hematoporphyrin as a diagnostic tool. A preliminary report of new techniques. Cancer 30: 1368–1372
35. Santamaria L, Prino G (1969) The photodynamic substances and their mechanism of action. Res Prog Org Biol Med Chem 1: 250–336
36. Tomson SH, Emmett EA, Fox SH (1974) Photodestruction of mouse epithelial tumours after acridine orange and argon laser. Cancer Res 34: 3124–3127
37. Vassar PS, Saunders AM, Gulling CFA (1960) Tetracycline fluorescence in malignant tumours and benign ulcers. Arch Pathol 69: 613–619
38. Winkelman J (1962) The distribution of tetraphenylporphine sulfonate in the tumour-bearing rat. Cancer Res 22: 589–596

Fluorescence Bronchoscopy
for Localizing Early Bronchial Cancer
and Carcinoma in Situ

O. J. Balchum, D. R. Doiron, A. E. Profio, and G. C. Huth

Los Angeles County-University of Southern California Medical Center,
Pulmonary Disease Section, Department of Medicine, California, CA, USA

Introduction

The detection, diagnosis, and aggressive treatment of lung cancer in its intrabronchial
or preinvasive phase has been shown to result in 5-year survival rates of over
70%−80% [16, 19, 29]. In the case of carcinoma in situ, resection may result in
prolonged survival and possibly cure [4]. In contrast, stage I lung cancer is of the
invasive type and includes lesions that have already extended to the ipsilateral hilar
lymph nodes; the 5-year survival at this stage is at best about 40%−50%. In small
peripheral lung cancers (less than 3.0 cm in diameter), visible on chest X-ray but
without hilar lymph node involvement, 5-year survival can be up to 60% [18].
The goal of physicians, therefore, must be the diagnosis of *preinvasive* lung cancer in
patients at high risk. High risk patients include heavy cigarette smokers who have
smoked one package per day or more for 20 years or longer, particularly those over age
45 years. Patients at particularly high risk are heavy smokers who also have symptoms
or signs related to lung cancer and especially include smokers who have also been
occupationally exposed to asbestos, uranium mining, coke oven emissions, nickel, and
chromates, which are known industrial carcinogens.
The detection of early lung cancer in its occult or semioccult phase is by sputum
cytology for malignant cells. Radiologically occult lung cancer is revealed when the
chest X-ray is negative, but the sputum analysis is positive for malignant cells. In
semioccult disease, the patient also has symptoms and/or signs which may be related to
bronchial cancer, but which remain radiologically occult or nonspecific. These include
increased or unexplained cough, blood streaking of sputum, a slowly resolving
pneumonia or lung infiltrate, obstructive pneumonitis, localized hyperlucency or
atelectasis of lung segments on chest X-ray, whether fleeting or persistent. Neither
these nor any other X-ray appearance can be considered to be specific for lung cancer;
however, a malignant sputum cytology is specific. The examination of sputum for
malignant cells is, therefore, essential in diagnosing early lung cancer. For high
accuracy and reliability, adequate sputum collections and concentration and
processing methods are essential to retrieve sputum cells efficiently [23]. Not only
spontaneous deep-cough morning specimens, collected directly into 50% alcohol −
2% Carbowax fixative, but nebulized water aerosol induced sputum samples are
required [18, 23]. Specimens should be multiple (five or more) in highly suspect
individuals. High accuracy of diagnosis can be achieved (95%), with few false positives

Recent Results in Cancer Research, Vol. 82
© Springer-Verlag Berlin · Heidelberg 1982

(less than 1%). Accurate diagnosis particularly requires cytological reading and interpretation in competent and experienced hands [6]. Since lung cancers may be peripheral or obstruct a bronchus, sputum cytology may fail to reveal malignant cells in about 15% of lung cancers. Chest X-ray, therefore, is also required for diagnosis of early lung cancers in highly suspect patients, but alone they are not sufficient.

Technically the chest X-rays must be of high quality exposure and contrast. Reading and interpretation must be in experienced hands to achieve a high sensitivity for detecting small, localized infiltrates or nodules of nonspecific appearance. Serial comparison films with evaluation of all previous X-rays and double readings are required to recognize the first visualization of a small X-ray abnormality that may be lung cancer.

Since there can be a long natural history of slow progression of bronchial cancer over many years, the physician applying these two clinical tools has both the opportunity and the obligation to detect lung cancer early in his high risk patients.

Saccomanno has shown by chronological sputum cytology in smokers and uranium miners that there is a prolonged and slow progression of metaplasia of the bronchial mucosal cells over as long as 10−15 years [18, 25]. This serial progression is from metaplasia through phases of mild, moderate, then marked atypia (premalignant), and finally to carcinoma in situ. The subsequent stage of microinvasive cancer is reached over an interval averaging 4−5 years. There is therefore a "golden period" in which preinvasive lung cancer remaining confined to the bronchus can be detected by sputum cytology and in which patient cure rate by resection can reach over 90% [30].

Once the diagnosis of early or occult lung cancer has been obtained by sputum cytology, the site of the tumor must be localized within the tracheobronchial tree. Bronchial cancer may be present at more than one site.

Small bronchial cancers are located by routine fiberoptic bronchoscopy in less than 50% of instances. Even repeated bronchoscopies over a period of time commonly fail. This problem has frustrated physicians to the point of doubting the value of sputum cytology in the early diagnosis of lung cancer.

One approach to the problem of localization of small bronchial cancers has been to perform fiberoptic bronchoscopic examination under general anesthesia, requiring several hours for inspection of proximal and distal bronchi, including segmental and subsegmental branchings throughout the lungs. Search is for visible mucosal and bronchial lesions for specific diagnosis by bronchial brushings and bite biopsies. These can be negative so that carcinoma in situ is still not localized. Such cases require extensive bronchial brushings of 30−40 or more lung segments and subsegments, as well as blind biopsies of the spurs. Even in experienced hands not more than 50% of occult tumors are initially localized, so that additional (up to five) extensive bronchoscopic examinations with multiple brushings may be required to locate finally the site of the lesions [26].

A new approach that we are evaluating is fluorescence bronchoscopy. This procedure is based on the use of hematoporphyrin derivative which is accumulated and retained in malignant tissue and emits a red fluorescence upon excitation by violet light. Lipson et al. [12] devised a mercury arc lamp as the source of violet light and a quartz fiber was used to carry the light into the rigid bronchoscope. Endobronchial cancers were visualized by their fluorescence [8, 13], but the rigid instruments limited inspection to the proximal and larger bronchi. With the advent of fiberoptic bronchoscopy, there was renewed interest in this method. A fiberoptic bronchoscope was devised with enhanced capability for transmission of violet light [27], but consistent and reliable localization of small lung tumors could not be achieved. This instrument, with the addition of an image intensifier and new arc lamp system, was used by Doiron et al. [5] and later by Balchum et al. (unpublished work) to visualize small lung cancers by their fluorescing images. A second type of instrument developed at the Mayo Clinic employs a photoelectric fluorescence energy detector that generates a sound signal when the emission of fluorescence is above background and within the visual field of the bronchoscope, although no fluorescing images were visualized [10]. This apparatus has been used successfully in detecting carcinoma in situ when only subtle or even no apparent mucosal abnormality was visible on ordinary white light inspection [3].

Our efforts have been directed toward developing improved instrumentation and methods for the visualization and recording of fluorescing bronchial cancers. The basic instrument, recently described by Profio et al. [21], essentially consists of a fiberoptic bronchoscope, image intensifier and a laser light source to produce monochromatic violet light of the proper wavelength to excite hematoporphyrin. The violet light is conducted via a small quartz fiber inserted through the channel of the bronchoscope. The tracheobronchial tree can be inspected first with white light and then with violet light. Small and even invisible bronchial cancers can be located by their fluorescence [9] for confirmation by brush and bite biopsies.

In this article we report the results of the first 38 patients we have investigated by this method and discuss the accuracy of fluorescence bronchoscopy by determining true positive, true negative, false positive, and false negative results.

Methods

The initial patients selected had sputum positive for malignant cells. Most had lung infiltrates and/or hilar enlargement on chest X-ray. A few had symptoms and chest X-rays suggestive of lung cancer but negative sputum cytology. As the study proceeded, patients with occult bronchial cancer and others not suspected to have lung cancer were studied.

Detailed explanation of the study was given to the patients, both verbally and in writing. Indications and alternatives were explained. Signed informed consent was then obtained.

The hematoporphyrin derivative (Hpd) employed was provided by Dr. Thomas J. Dougherty, Roswell Park Memorial Hospital, Buffalo, New York, in 30-ml serum capped bottles (sterile and pyrogen free). It was kept frozen until used, when it was allowed to liquefy by gentle warming.

Hpd was injected 72 h before fluorescence bronchoscopy at a dose of 2 mg/kg as a slow, pulsed push over 5–10 min into the tubing of a fast running intravenous solution to avoid local extravasation and venous irritation.

Workup included a complete blood count, white blood cell and platelet counts, prothrombin time, an SMA 12 blood chemistry panel, and urinalysis. An arterial blood gas, electrocardiogram, and usually a spirogram were obtained. History for clinical evidence of bleeding diatheses was specifically evaluated. These observations and measurements were repeated weekly for 3–4 weeks.

During Hpd injection and over the following hour, changes in vital signs and subjective local and systemic symptoms were monitored, with close observation of each patient for the next 3–4 h.

Patients were kept from being exposed to outside light, sunlight, and light entering windows. They were cautioned not to stand at a window or be close to reading lamps for an extended period of time. Upon leaving the hospital, verbal and written instructions and directions emphasized the continued need to avoid direct window light, close reading lamps, and particularly outside light and sunlight exposure over the next 4 weeks. A sunscreen cream was provided to cover the hands, face, forehead, and neck when outside. Patients were also instructed to wear a hat and a long-sleeved shirt, blouse, or jacket when outside over this period.

The fluorescence bronchoscope system used was that previously described by Profio and Doiron [21]. It consisted of a violet krypton ion laser as an exciting source and a first generation image intensifier for visualizing the emitted low-level red fluorescence through the bronchoscope. The laser is a Spectra-Physics Model 164-11/265 continuous ion laser with a typical output before filtering of 240 mW in three lines at 406.7 nm (36%), 413.1 nm (60%), and 415.4 nm (4%). The fluorescence exciting light is delivered to the bronchus via a fused quartz step-index fiber (0.8 mm outer diameter), inserted into the small biopsy channel of a dual channel Olympus bronchoscope, Model BF-2T. The image intensifier is coupled to the standard ocular of the bronchoscope with a transfer lens giving a 2.4 times magnification. Secondary filters between the bronchoscope ocular and the intensifier block the reflected violet light and pass the emitted fluorescence red light. The intensifier is a Varo model 8858 three stage intensifier with an extended red photocathode (S20VR) and green P-20 output phosphor. It has a minimum luminous gain of 30,000 Fl/Fc. The low level red fluorescence image is thereby converted to a bright green image more easily visualized by the bronchoscopist. Fluorescing sites were viewed first using a broad-band secondary filter (620–730 nm), and then a narrow-band filter (670–720 nm). The former gives a brighter image while the latter has a better signal-to-background ratio. Photographs of the fluorescence image are taken by a 35-mm single-lens reflex camera attached to the image intensifier ocular, allowing direct visualization during photography through the camera. This system is extremely sensitive and capable of visualizing an Hpd concentration of 0.1 µg/ml in a well 100 µm (0.1 mm) in depth and 1.5 mm in width.

It must be emphasized that the violet irradiance of the system (12 mW/cm^2) is insufficient to cause significant heat or photodynamic reaction that might damage the tumor or the normal bronchial tissue.

Bronchoscopy was carried out under local anesthesia of the upper and lower airways after premedication with atropine and meperidine hydrochloride. As studies proceeded, a Cardens oral endotracheal tube was consistently used [2]. This was to enable withdrawal of the bronchoscope after each brushing of each site. The brush (Meditech, 3 mm diameter bristles) was drawn up to near the tip but not into the channel of the bronchoscope, in order not to wipe off mucus or secretions. Smears were immediately made on Dakin frosted slides that were promptly immersed into 95% alcohol. Bite biopsies with Olympus or Machida forceps were immediately put into 10% neutral formalin. An Olympus CLV light source was used for white light illumination.

Thorough inspection of the upper and then lower airways was carried out under white light to the subsegmental level. The orifices and initial extent of the subsegmental bronchi in each lobe of the lungs were visualized. Next, inspection of the entire tracheobronchial tree was carried out using violet light to visualize fluorescence. Examination for areas of fluorescence over the main carina and the spurs between lobar, segmental, and subsegmental bronchi was carefully done, with attempts to use several angles of incident exciting violet light by manipulation of the tip of the fiberoptic bronchoscope. The lips or margins of bronchial orifices were also carefully inspected, as well as the walls. As studies proceeded, bronchoscopy could be effectively carried out using either the broad-band or the narrow-band filter under the illumination provided by the diffuse background fluorescent light from bronchial tissues.

Records of findings included sound/cassette taping of the entire procedure, both by the bronchoscopist (O.J.B.) and separately by the physicist regulating the laser violet light source and in charge of photography (D.R.D.). The latter also recorded sites of visible and of fluorescing lesions and the sequence and exposures of photographs taken. In addition and highly useful were written records which included one separate structured sheet each for white light bronchoscopic findings, fluorescent light bronchoscopic findings, sites of brush biopsies, and sites of bite biopsies. The sheets listed all the structures from the pharynx, pyriform sinuses, larynx, trachea, etc., down to the segmental bronchi of each lobe.

A great deal of effort and a large number of trials were devoted to photographing under white light and under fluorescent light those sites with visible lesions that fluoresced, as well as normal appearing sites that showed only a background fluorescence level. Various types of 35-mm high-speed color and black and white films were used. A series of exposure times were employed. Both slides and enlarged color prints were tried. We have finally selected Kodak Ektachrome 400 daylight film, EL 135-36, push developed to ASA 800 and a series of exposures of 1/8, 1/15, and 1/30 of a second to produce color slides. Fluorescence photos were taken at 1/4, 1/8, 1/15, 1/30, and 1/60 of a second to assure adequate exposure and to extend the visualized span of recorded images.

The weight of the camera (Olympus OM-1 and OM-2) when attached to the bronchoscope for white light photographing was counterbalanced by a boom. The image intensifier and camera contributed additional weight. It was found that greater stability was required than that afforded by a balanced boom. After trial by two methods of rigid support apparatus, the final support was constructed using a commercially available, very stable, camera monostand. This employs, on the rigid vertical monostand, an arm which can be extended horizontally up to 3 feet (if required) and is counterbalanced. From the end of this horizontal arm, a vertical support, 14 inches long, consisting of two ball-joints in tandem, terminates in a ring through which the image intensifier could slide and then be fixed. This stand allows for easy positioning in three dimensions of the image intensifier with the attached bronchoscope and camera.

The details of apparatus, equipment, and construction are important because complete bronchoscopic inspection, white light and fluorescence photography, and brush and bite biopsies must all be carried out within the limits of the time allowed by local anesthesia. At present, the total time required is approximately $1^{1}/_{2}$ h, especially when several fluorescing sites are detected which must be photographed, brushed, and bite biopsied. We also photograph, brush, and bite biopsy any subtle abnormal sites that do not fluoresce, as well as for comparison sites that appear normal under white and violet light. The actual fluorescence examination takes approximately 20 min.

Types of Fluorescence Visualized

Visible endobronchial (mucosal) tumors showed *positive localized fluorescence* that was bright and had high contrast to surrounding structures (Fig. 1). In a few instances, there was diffuse fluorescence or a shield-shaped area of less intense fluorescence surrounding a bronchial orifice, but that was clearly in contrast with the background fluorescence of adjacent normal structures. This appearance was termed *positive diffuse fluorescence* (Fig. 2). Areas appearing normal (under white light) were seen that showed distinct positive fluorescence, either a small area of localized fluorescence or a larger, collar-shaped area of diffuse but distinct fluorescence. When it could not be decided whether positive fluorescence (either localized or diffuse) was being visualized, these areas were called *equivocal or indeterminate fluorescence* (Fig. 3).

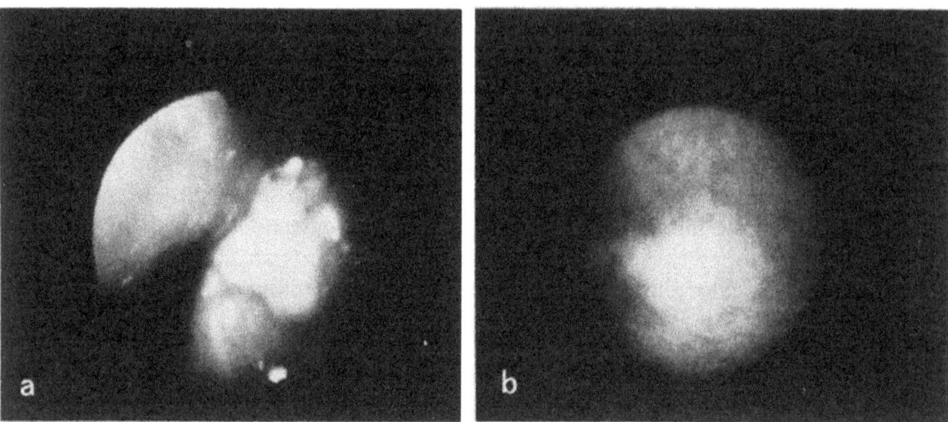

Fig. 1a, b. Positive localized fluorescence. **a** Visible endobronchial cancer in RUL bronchus *(white light)*. **b** Positive localized fluorescence *(fluorescent light)*. Note high contrast relative to area of background fluorescence above

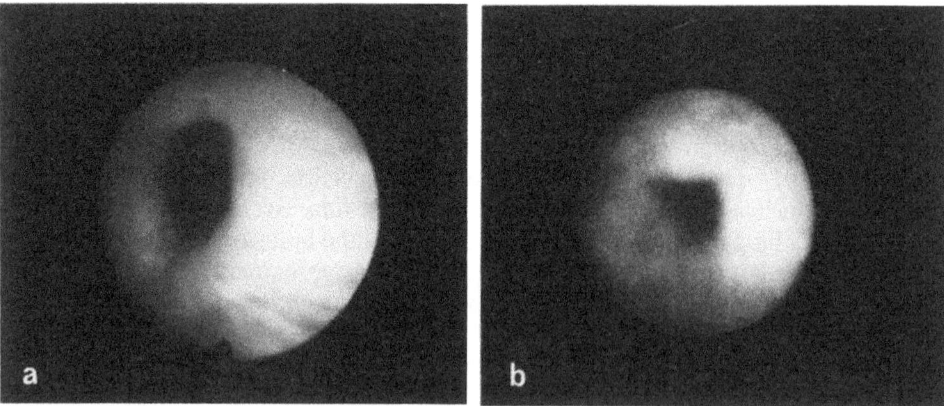

Fig. 2a, b. Positive diffuse fluorescence. **a** Visible area of mucosal thickening at lip of RLL bronchus *(white light)*. **b** Positive diffuse fluorescence of this area under fluorescent light. Note high contrast relative to background fluorescing area at lower left

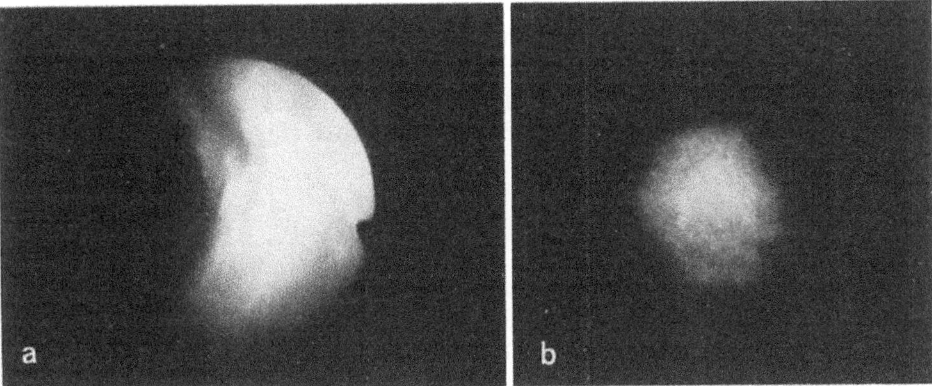

Fig. 3a, b. Equivocal fluorescence − questionable. **a** Apparent mucosal irregularity visible under white light inspection. **b** Low contrast fluorescence that is equivocal or questionable − greater than background fluorescence of normal tissues but not of high contrast as seen in positive fluorescence

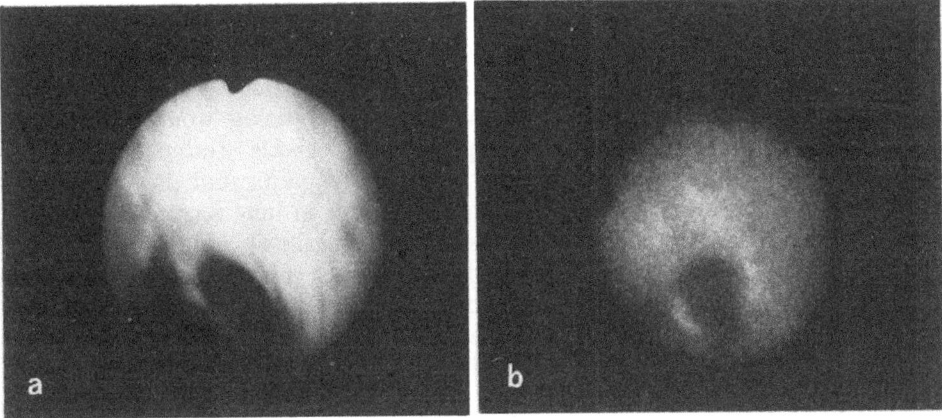

Fig. 4a, b. Negative fluorescence. **a** Whitish mucosa with irregularity in LLL bronchus under white light inspection. **b** Negative fluorescence: that of background of normal bronchial tissues. Clearly not positive nor equivocal

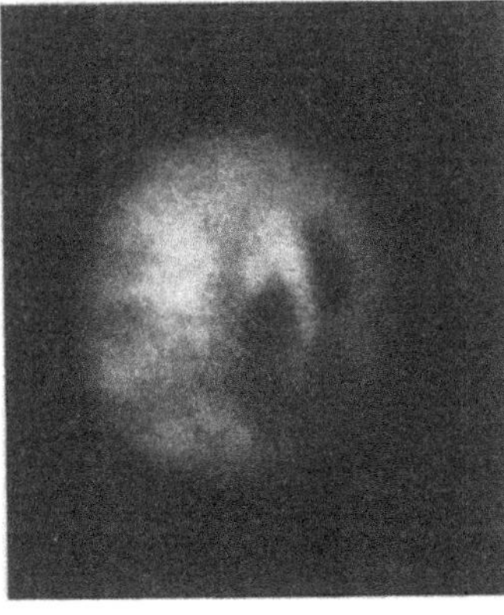

Fig. 5. Negative fluorescence (normal appearing area of RLL bronchus). This photograph taken under fluorescent light illustrates the details of bronchial mucosal structure and of bronchial orifices that can be visualized

The notion *negative fluorescence* was used when it was certain that neither positive nor equivocal fluorescence was seen and that the level of fluorescence clearly was that of background, i.e., that of the bronchial tree with normal appearance (Fig. 4). Quite intricate details of mucosal characteristics, of folds, and of bronchial orifices are visible under broad-band and narrow-band filter fluorescence (Fig. 5).

Diagnostic Accuracy of Fluorescence Bronchoscopy

The efficacy of fluorescence bronchoscopy is its ability to indicate the presence or the absence of bronchial cancer with a high degree of certainty.

Determining efficacy (predictive value) of fluorescence bronchoscopy is based on two key components: (1) determination of the disease status (cancer, other diseases, or normal) with a high degree of accuracy and confidence; and (2) determining whether or not there are positive fluorescing bronchial sites. To determine the accuracy (value) of fluorescence bronchoscopy, the "true" result or disease status at each fluorescing site and at other non-fluorescing sites must therefore be accurately known.

Determining the status of the disease with accuracy results from adequate methods of sputum collection and processing, the preparation of good smears, and accurate cytopathological reading and interpretation. For example, should a sputum be reported to show carcinoma cells, it would be reported as positive, and the patient would be suspected to have lung cancer. Should cytopathological interpretation be inaccurate and reported otherwise, then the status of the disease would be false. On the other hand, should the sputum be reported as "negative" (no malignant cells) owing to inadequate sputum collection or to faulty preparation and processing methods so that the majority of cells actually present in lung secretions were not retrieved, then the interpretation of the disease status again would be false. We have encountered both types of error. In this study, therefore, a great deal of effort has gone into instituting precise and valid methods of sputum collection, processing, and cytological interpretation for the accurate determination of disease status.

This precision is required for brush and bite biopsying at the time of bronchoscopy. The bronchoscopist must have the time and skill to obtain these samples from fluorescing and nonfluorescing sites as well as from visibly normal and abnormal (white light) sites, in order to establish the true nature of the disease status at all sites.

Either by direct smears or preferably from solutions into which the brush is introduced and the cells dislodged from it [24], the methods of smearing must be conducive to a good specimen. The smear must be thin and cover a small area for enhanced cytological interpretation.

In case of bronchial biopsies, was the intended site actually biopsied? In order not to miss the desired site, the number and the size of biopsies done at given sites must be adequate. Were serial sections examined and was the interpretation by the pathologist of high quality and accuracy? All of these conditions must be fulfilled with a high degree of confidence. Otherwise, the nature of the disease will be in error, confounding the determination of the efficacy of fluorescence bronchoscopy. It is clear that in addition to the fluorescence bronchoscopy instrumentation being tested and evaluated in the localization of early bronchial cancers and carcinoma in situ, that the other methods for evaluating disease status are of fundamental and equal importance.

Considerations in Determining the Presence of Positive Fluorescence

The major diagnostic component in the imaging of small bronchial cancer is contrast. In order to be recognized, the intensity of the fluorescing image of a small tumor must be greater than that of surrounding normal bronchial tissue. This is dependent upon the differences in Hpd concentrations between tumor and normal cells, the increased brightness due to the image intensifier and filters, and the intensity and uniformity of the incident violet light. For example, a bronchoscopic field should be uniformly illuminated with violet light without an interfering localized area of glare that obliterates details of structure. Image contrast and detail are, therefore, essential in providing diagnostic information [20].

Patterns of fluorescence must be recognized or perceived from the detail resulting from the contrast and resolution provided by the procedure, methods, and instruments [11, 20]. The "signal" or information from the fluorescing images must be comprehended and integrated by the bronchoscopist into diagnostic information, i.e., true fluorescence or not. Perception is increased by practice and experience from repeated fluorescent bronchoscopies. Accuracy of perception will probably be increased by alternately viewing bronchoscopic fields first with white light and then immediately with fluorescent light. Recognizing subtle abnormalities under white and fluorescent light is required to enhance the diagnosis of early lung cancer. A supplementary method of viewing bronchoscopic fields under white and fluorescent light is a television monitor with video tape recording. This will make interpretations of other observers promptly available at the time of bronchoscopy. The findings or patterns of images must then be interpreted. As a result of fluorescent bronchoscopy, there might be sites with positive, equivocal, or negative fluorescence. These require brushings and bite biopsies to establish whether cancer, other diseases, or normal tissue are present at the respective sites. Ultimately, gross and microscopic results from resected lobes or segments of lung will be required to determine the size, extent, and degree of microinvasion of cancer, the nature and extent of other diseases, and areas which can be clearly concluded to be normal.

To determine diagnostic or localizing power with accuracy and confidence depends on the accuracy of: (1) evaluation of disease status, and (2) fluorescence methods, instrumentation, and imaging as well as image perception at fluorescing sites.

Diagnostic Efficacy of Fluorescence Bronchoscopy

We use the following abbreviations (cf. Table 1):

TP: True Positive: Number or percentage of cancers with positive fluorescence: cancer correctly localized and diagnosed by fluorescence.

FP: False Positive: Number or percentage of noncancers (other disease, normal) with positive fluorescence: cancers incorrectly diagnosed by fluorescence.

FN: False Negative: Number or percentage of cancers incorrectly diagnosed as not to have cancer, because no fluorescence was seen.

TN: True Negative: Number or percentage of noncancers correctly diagnosed as noncancer (other disease, normal), since no fluorescence was seen.

The efficacy (efficiency) of a test procedure is expressed by four indices, each with a maximum value of 1.0 or 100%.

                                                                O. J. Balchum et al.

Table 1. Categories used in evaluating results of fluorescence bronchoscopy

Test result	True disease status		
	Cancer present	Cancer absent	
Positive fluorescence	TP	FP	TP + FP
Negative fluorescence	FN	TN	FN + TN
	TP + FN	FP + TN	TP + FP + FN + TN = S

Sensitivity. If the patient has lung cancer, how likely is a positive fluorescence at the cancer site?

Sensitivity = Positivity (positive fluorescence when cancer) = TP/(TP + FN).

Specificity. If there is no cancer, how likely is there to be positive fluorescence? Specificity = Negativity (no fluorescence when non-cancer, i.e., other diseases or normal) = TN/(TN + FP).

Rule in Cancer. If the patient has positive fluorescence (positive test), how likely is he to have lung cancer?

Accuracy for positive prediction or diagnosis (rule in) = True positives/Total positives = TP/(TP + FP).

Rule out Cancer. If the patient shows no fluorescence (negative test), how likely is he to have lung cancer?

Accuracy for negative prediction (rule out) = True negatives/Total negatives = TN/(FN + TN).

The predictive value of fluorescence bronchoscopy would have to be determined in an unselected or randomly selected population in order to answer the question: how accurately will it predict or diagnose the presence or absence of bronchial cancer? Predictive value is determined by the incidence of FN results in patients *with* bronchial cancer, by the incidence of FP results in subjects without bronchial cancer and by the prevalence of the disease [7, 22].

Ultimately, determination of predictive or diagnostic value will require the evaluation of subjects who are free of disease (normal), subjects who are free of bronchial cancer but have other bronchial diseases, and subjects who have lung cancer. A broad spectrum of patients with lung cancer must be evaluated by fluorescence bronchoscopy in order to determine its accuracy and power for negative prediction (rule out cancer). This spectrum must particularly include subjects with occult lung cancer (chest X-ray negative, sputum positive for malignant cells) and those having small visible and nonvisible bronchial cancer sites on white light bronchoscopy.

The initial evaluations of a test procedure are usually sensitivity and specificity. The last two indices (rule in, rule out) depend not only on sensitivity and specificity but also on prevalence of the disease. Prevalence = the percentage of the total number of subjects examined who have the disease = (TP + FN)/S, where S = TP + FP + TN + FN.

The clinician's diagnostic goals are to rule in (diagnose positive) and rule out (exclude) the presence of a disease. To rule in or diagnose lung cancer, fluorescence bronchoscopy should have a high accuracy for positive prediction. This requires few FP and thus high specificity. A broad range of patients *without* lung cancer (other disease, normal) must be studied to determine the accuracy of positive prediction.

To rule out or exclude lung cancer, fluorescence bronchoscopy should have a high accuracy for negative prediction (not lung cancer). This requires few FN and thus a high sensitivity. To determine the accuracy of negative prediction requires a broad range of patients *with* lung cancer, including very early (in situ) and early (locally microinvasive) intrabronchial cancer, as well as instances of invasive cancer including spread over a broad range of extension to ipsilateral hilum, to mediastinal lymph nodes and finally with dissemination to other organ systems.

Efficiency of fluorescence bronchoscopy = the percentage of all results that are true results, whether positive or negative, that is: Efficiency = (TP + TN)/S.

The prevalence rate (ratio of number of patients with lung cancer to the total number of patients examined) affects the predictive or diagnostic value of a test, regardless of its sensitivity and specificity:

$$\text{Predictive value} = \frac{(\text{Prevalence})\ (\text{Sensitivity})}{(\text{Prev.})\ (\text{Sensitiv.}) + (1\text{-Prev.})\ (1\text{-Specif.})}\ .$$

The greater the prevalence of lung cancer in the group of patients studied, the greater will be the predictive value of positive fluorescence for lung cancer. When prevalence is 50% or more, the predictive value of a test can be 95% or more.

To evaluate fluorescence bronchoscopy, therefore, it must be determined whether it is highly sensitive and whether it yields false negative results and why. This must be decided on the basis of the lung cancer pathology, including extent, location and cell type. Fluorescence bronchoscopy should be positive in patients with early or intrabronchial lung cancer (carcinoma in situ or mucosal cancer plaque and cancer, yet localized to bronchus, but with microinvasion through basement membrane), as well as invasive cancer that has metastasized to the hilum. Fluorescence bronchoscopy must have a high sensitivity for diagnosing lung cancer in asymptomatic patients and also when there are acute symptoms (recent blood streaking of sputum) or chronic symptoms (atelectasis), over a broad range of severity.

Fluorescence bronchoscopy must be evaluated in patients with coexisting other diseases that might make it falsely negative. For example, the edema and excessive mucus of chronic obstructive bronchitis may obscure visualizing and perceiving small positive fluorescing sites. In turn, patients should be studied with diseases that could yield false positive results, such as inflammatory bronchial diseases that may produce localized bronchial alterations and mucosal changes that might fluoresce or be perceived to fluoresce. Decision as to whether the patient has a lung cancer or other diseases or is normal may require long-term follow-up evaluation.

Ideally, the physician performing fluorescence bronchoscopy should be unaware of the status of sputum cytology, i.e., not know whether the patient has bronchial cancer or not. Whether there are positive fluorescing sites and whether sputum cytology shows tumor cells should be determined by totally independent investigators. Otherwise, workup bias may result from either a positive or negative test. Positive fluorescence may make the clinician look more intensely for lung cancer than if it were negative. Negative fluorescence could cause the diagnosis of lung cancer to be missed because additional tests were not done.

Ultimately, cost-benefit analysis should be considered [28]. This should include the cost of equipment, technical difficulties in the use of fluorescence bronchoscopy apparatus, problems of mechanical variability, and the training required for expertise in fluorescence bronchoscopy. The value and costs of methods used for recording fluorescence images must also be included. Of vital importance in estimating benefits are not only associated risks and morbidity, but particularly the clinical benefits to the patient from the diagnosis provided that leads to a high cure rate by the surgical resection of early lung cancer. Questions to be answered are: Does fluorescence bronchoscopy for localization of preinvasive lung cancer and of early local microinvasive cancer appreciably increase life span after treatment by present curative methods (surgical resection)? When the latter is not possible, do new methods of localized therapy (photoradiation therapy) provide measurable benefit to patients?

The costs and benefits of localizing early (preinvasive) lung cancer by fluorescence bronchoscopy must be compared with those resulting from repeated routine bronchoscopy and with those of extended bronchoscopy (multiple brushings/biopsies under general anesthesia). Included must be the negative benefits to the patient of diagnosing cancer when it is already invasive (stage I or more advanced), and the costs of and morbidity due to present palliative therapies such as radiation and chemotherapy. Reports of the costs and benefits of present methods and therapy of advanced (invasive) lung cancer have not as yet been published, but a model has been suggested [17].

Results

Hematoporphyrin Derivative Toxicity and Skin Photosensitivity

Fifty intravenous injections of Hpd were given to 38 patients at a dose of 2 mg/kg without any localized or systemic toxicity or allergic reactions. No changes in vital signs or any symptoms, either immediate or late, have been observed following Hpd injection. No hematological, liver and renal functions, or urinalysis abnormalities were observed which could be attributed to Hpd.

No significant skin photosensitivity reactions occurred. There were three instances of mild sunburn, due to patients not strictly adhering to the precautions and protective measures in which they were instructed. These were exposures to direct, outside sunlight for periods of approximately 15 min to 1 h. All sunlight exposures occurred within 2 weeks after injection. A prickling sensation of the skin was felt, followed several hours later by mild erythema and edema of the forehead and cheeks. These three mild sunburns were self-limiting and disappeared within 24 h without treatment. They occurred in a black, a Chinese, and an Italian patient with a dark complexion. It is evident that even very dark skin does not in itself offer enough protection against the skin photosensitivity induced by hematoporphyrin derivative.

Instrumentation and Laser Light Source

There were no notable problems with the power supply or the laser light source, which functioned well consistently. The quartz fiber was inserted to the tip of the

Table 2. Positive fluorescence at same sites in three patients who underwent fluorescence bronchoscopy twice

1) Small cell carcinoma − Spur LU/LL division
2) Adenocarcinoma − RUL, RML, LUL
3) Squamous cell carcinoma − RUL, apical segment
                                             RML, anterior lip
     Reproducible for main histologic types

two-channel bronchoscope. Initially at times a "hot spot" was present, i.e., a concentrated round glare occupying about one-quarter of the field, with a lesser but adequate intensity of illumination in the remaining area. This was remedied by slightly adjusting the distance of the fiber tip to extend its relation to the end of the bronchoscope channel. The divergence of the fiber was later increased to a 40° C field of view by forcing the light into higher optical modes of transmission in the fiber. Occasionally, the tip of the fiber became occluded with mucus deposit so that violet light intensity was inadequate; then the quartz fiber had to be withdrawn and its tip cleaned.

A sufficient violet light illumination was provided so that fluorescence intensity with the broad-band filter and the narrow-band filter allowed visual outlining of the normal structures by their "background" fluorescence. This broad-band background fluorescence is caused by the violet light exciting normal tissues. Skill was developed so that the entire tracheobronchial tree could be inspected under the intensity of fluorescence provided by either filter. The thin edges of normal spurs were often bright. Mucosal folds were well outlined when present, as in inflammation due to chronic bronchitis. Fine details of mucosal structure could be seen (Fig. 5). Localized mucus deposits on the mucosa did not frequently give difficulty or interfere in identifying true fluorescence.

Reproducibility of Fluorescence Bronchoscopy and Histologic Types of Cancer

Three patients underwent fluorescence bronchoscopy twice, about 2 weeks apart. Table 2 illustrates that the specific fluorescent bronchoscopy method and instrumentation used give reproducible results, as the same sites fluoresced in each instance in the three patients.

All three main histologic types of bronchial cancer (squamous cell, adenocarcinoma, and small cell undifferentiated carcinoma) were found to fluoresce reproducibly. Tumor was also observed in another patients with large cell undifferentiated carcinoma.

True Positive Fluorescence

Twenty-two patients were regarded as true positives, showing fluorescing sites which were demonstrated to be carcinoma by brush and bite biopsies. Twelve patients had squamous cell carcinoma, four adenocarcinoma, two small cell, and one large cell undifferentiated carcinoma, and three had malignant cells that could not be classified.

Sputum cytology showed cancer cells in 18 but was negative in four patients. Chest X-rays were normal in three patients, all of whom had malignant cells in sputum and therefore had occult lung cancer. In 13 patients chest X-rays were suggestive of lung cancer. Of these, 10 had visible endobronchial main stem or lobar bronchial masses of varying sizes, and in one the cancer lesion was in the trachea. Two had subtle changes consisting of irregularity or of a whitish aspect of the mucosa over a spur. Of four patients showing nonspecific infiltrates on chest X-ray, three had visible mucosal masses; one had non, with only a whitish mucosal coat covering a spur. Of two patients with atelectasis, one had a mucosal mass and the other a whitish mucosal coat over a spur. In three patients with normal chest X-rays, one showed a mass in the left main stem bronchus, one had a small area of mucosal irregularity over a spur, and the third had widening of a spur without visible mucosal abnormality or lesion.

Positive fluorescence was seen in all 22 patients. Fourteen patients had one site, seven had two sites, and one had three sites of positive fluorescence. In a patient with two fluorescing sites, one site showed positive and the other equivocal fluorescence. The latter, the only equivocal site seen in these 22 patients, was at a focus of hemorrhagic mucosa which was normal on biopsy.

There were 28 sites of positive fluorescence confirmed to be carcinoma by brush and bite biopsies in these 22 true positive fluorescence patients. Of these 28 sites, 15 were squamous cell carcinoma, five adenocarcinoma, two small cell, one large cell undifferentiated carcinoma, and in five the carcinoma could not be classified. One site that showed positive fluorescence was carcinoma in situ on biopsy.

There was one false negative site, in that no fluorescence was seen but bronchial brushings showed carcinoma in situ. There were three false positive sites, since positive fluorescence was seen at these areas but brush and bite biopsies did not reveal cancer. They showed normal mucosa, chronic inflammation with squamous metaplasia, and chronic inflammation, respectively. There were 20 true negative sites.

True Positive Occult Lung Cancer

Localization of the site(s) of small bronchial cancer is difficult by white light bronchoscopy, even when careful extended inspection and multiple brush and bite biopsies are carried out [26]. Smokers, chronic bronchitis, and patients with chronic obstructive pulmonary disease (COPD) may show a number of bronchial sites at which there is slight visible abnormality, such as irregularity or granularity of the mucosa or small white mucosal patches over spurs or at the orifices of bronchi. The following case illustrates the advantages of fluorescence bronchoscopy in directly locating the cancer site for brush and bite biopsies in occult carcinoma when there are several sites with subtle abnormalities visible on white light inspection. The patient was a 67-year-old man who had been a uranium miner for 28 years and smoked $1-1\frac{1}{2}$ packages of cigarettes per day for 30 years. He had moderately severe COPD with lung hyperinflation on chest X-ray and on spirometry. Serial sputum cytology studies by Dr. G. Saccomanno revealed carcinoma in situ in four samples. When he underwent fluorescence bronchoscopy, in May, malignant cells were seen in three sputum samples. Bronchoscopy revealed a small area of mucosal irregularity at the entrance of the lateral basilar segment of the RLL[1] which showed positive localized fluorescence

---

1 RLL, right lower lobe; RML, right middle lobe; RUL, right upper lobe; LLL, left lower lobe; LML, left middle lobe; LUL, left upper lobe

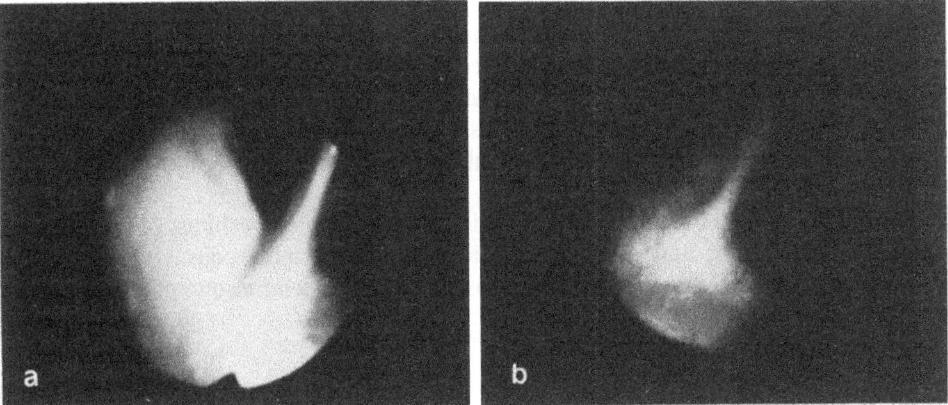

Fig. 6a, b. Carcinoma in situ showing true positive fluorescence. Patient with occult lung cancer (chest X-ray negative, sputum positive for malignant cells). **a** Spur between lateral and posterior basilar bronchi of RLL, indicating possible mucosal thickening at its base under white light inspection. **b** Positive localized fluorescence over base of spur

(Fig. 6). The subsegmental bronchi distal to this site appeared normal with no areas of positive fluorescence seen. Brushings at the site of fluorescence showed carcinoma cells. The RUL brushings showed a small, white protrusion on its anterior lip. The LUL bronchus had a small area of irregular mucosa, as did the entrance to the anterior-medial segmental bronchus of the LLL. The posterior and lateral segmental bronchi of the LLL appeared normal. None of these sites fluoresced and brush biopsies showed normal mucosa negative for tumor cells.

True Negative

Seven patients did not show any area of positive or equivocal fluorescence. They are regarded as true negatives as sputum samples and bronchoscopic brush and bite biopsies did not reveal carcinoma, and since fluorescence bronchoscopy was entirely negative. Two of these seven patients were examined by bronchoscopy because of slight hemoptysis and had localized bronchiectasis secondary to previous pneumonia. Two had upper lung field densities, and one had bilateral upper lobe infiltrates; in each case bronchoscopy was performed for diagnosis. Two had previous sputum cytology obtained and read elsewhere as malignant, but on review showed moderate atypia.

Sputum samples were negative in five, and two showed moderate atypia. Five or more sputum samples were obtained before bronchoscopy from each patient. In the three patients with negative chest X-rays, 10–18 pre- and postbronchoscopy sputum samples were obtained. Two other patients showed small infiltrates in the RUL; another had a small subpleural density in the left apex ultimately diagnosed as tuberculosis on bronchoscopic biopsy. The remaining patient had small patchy infiltrates in both upper lobes.

White light bronchoscopy of these seven patients revealed no abnormalities suggestive of carcinoma. Of three patients with normal chest X-rays, two had no bronchial abnormalities. One had granularity of the mucosa in the RLL bronchus, just proximal to the medial basilar segmental orifice. The fourth patient (RUL infiltrate) had slight concentric narrowing of the RUL bronchus but no mucosal abnormality. The fifth patient had a distorted spur, not thickened, between the right posterior and lateral segmental bronchi. The sixth patient showed only whitish plaque over several spurs. The last patient had slight bronchial mucosal irregularity in the RUL, RLL, and LLL bronchi. None of these areas with subtle abnormalities fluoresced, nor did areas that appeared normal.

Extensive brushings, brush and bite biopsies, and bronchial washings of the areas of visible abnormalities, and other areas, did not reveal cancer cells.

Biopsies showed normal mucosa, except in one patient in whom squamous metaplasia was found.

False Positives

There were nine patients considered to be false positives in that sites of positive fluorescence did not reveal carcinoma on brush and bite biopsies.

The main cause for these false positives is regarded to be inadequate brush and bite biopsies at the numerous sites demanded in this study. There is a limit to the duration of good local anesthesia before coughing and discomfort begin which makes biopsying difficult and therefore probably inadequate. Achieving thorough and efficient bronchoscopic inspection under white and fluorescent light took practice with sequential revision of methods and adaptations of equipment. This took up anesthesia time. A second area concentrated upon was achieving the maximal retrieval of cells by brush biopsy specimens and the proper preparation of smears from the brush specimens. Quality control measures to achieve accurate cytopathological interpretation were instituted.

A second cause of false positives that still has to be further investigated is that localized areas of bronchial mucosal inflammation or metaplasia may in some instances retain Hpd and cause positive fluorescence.

Our first patient with false positive fluorescence illustrates false positivity due to inability to retrieve adequate diagnostic material. In this case, the bronchial biopsy had to be done blindly since the left main stem bronchus was concentrically narrowed to 10% of its usual diameter. The patient had sputum positive for poorly differentiated squamous carcinoma. Chest X-rays showed a LUL infiltrate. Brushings and biopsy at a previous bronchoscopy had also failed to retrieve specimens that revealed carcinoma. A mass of widened spur between the left upper and lower division was seen to be positively fluorescent through the small remaining orifice of the left main stem bronchus, which could not be entered with the tip of the bronchoscope. Inserting the biopsy forceps completely occluded vision, so that biopsies were blind and failed to retrieve tumor tissue. Bronchial washings from the left lung revealed adenocarcinoma (as did the resected lung). Since positive bronchial brushings and/or biopsies were the criteria set for positive diagnosis of cancer, this patient was regarded as false positive.

The next two patients were evaluated because of sputum cytology diagnosed elsewhere as highly suspicious for carcinoma. These slides were later reviewed and diagnosed as moderate atypia. Chest X-rays were negative in one and showed a 1-cm RUL nodule unchanged over 3 years in the other patient. On bronchoscopy, the first patient showed no mucosal lesions but had whitish patches at the orifices of the RUL, RML,

RLL, LUL, and lingula. Positive fluorescence was noted in the RUL bronchus over the RML/RLL spur, and over the main carina (the latter appeared normal to white light inspection). Bronchial brushings showed mild atypia. Biopsy of the main carina showed mild squamous metaplasia, and those of RUL and the RML/RLL spur showed normal bronchial mucosa and were negative for tumor.

The above two patients as well as the next two patients may represent either positive fluorescence at sites of bronchial inflammation or failure to retrieve accurate and adequate brush and bite biopsy specimens. One had chest X-rays showing hyperinflated lungs and 16 specimens negative for malignant cells. An area of diffuse positive fluorescence was seen in the RUL bronchus, the mucosa of which showed slight irregularity on white light inspection. Bronchial brushings of this area showed mild metaplasia and biopsy did not reveal cancer cells. The other patient had infiltrates in the RUL and RLL with one sputum sample showing moderate atypia. Positive fluorescence was seen over the spur between the RML and RLL, and at the entrance of the RLL bronchus. Brushings showed squamous metaplasia and did not reveal cancer cells: biopsies showed squamous metaplasia with focal atypia. A third site in the anterior segment of the RUL showed equivocal fluorescence. Bronchial brushings were negative for tumor cells and biopsy showed chronic inflammation.

Two additional patients with false positive fluorescence bronchoscopies had rounded peripheral densities on chest X-rays; sputum was negative for tumor cells. In one, bronchoscopy was negative except for a small area of whitish mucosa in the RUL bronchus that showed positive fluorescence. Brushings were negative and biopsy showed chronic inflammation. In the other patient, two small areas of positive fluorescence were seen over the spur between the anterior and posterior segments of the RUL. Bronchial brushing and bite biopsies were negative for tumor cells and showed chronic inflammation. Transthoracic needle aspiration of the peripheral density in the first patient showed poorly differentiated carcinoma, and in the second poorly differentiated squamous cell carcinoma. In these patients, either biopsy of the sites of fluorescence was inaccurate or inadequate or perhaps sites of chronic inflammation or metaplasia were fluorescing.

The last two false positive patients were uranium miners and smokers who had occult carcinoma with negative chest X-rays and sputa positive for malignant cells (carcinoma in situ). The first had no endobronchial abnormalities; the spur between the RML and RLL bronchus appeared to be slightly irregular and thickened and showed positive fluorescence. Brushings were negative and bite biopsies showed squamous metaplasia and chronic inflammation. The second patient had two sites of positive localized fluorescence. The first was in the LLL where there was a small area of mucosal thickening. Brushings were negative and biopsies showed chronic inflammation. Bronchial washings showed atypical abnormal cells but were not interpreted to be cancer cells. The other area showed diffuse positive fluorescence over the lip of the RML bronchus. Both brushings and washings showed atypical cells, but bite biopsies did not reveal carcinoma. The cause of false positivity in both patients with occult lung cancer was attributed to inadequate or inaccurate retrieval of specimens from the positive fluorescing sites.

In these nine patients regarded as having false positive fluorescence, there were 16 false positive sites, since there was positive fluorescence but no carcinoma was revealed on brush and bite biopsies. There were 12 true negative sites, those showing no fluorescence and that were negative for carcinoma. There were no false negative or true positive sites.

Five of these false positive patients most likely had lung cancer, in two of whom it was occult. In the reamining four false positive patients, false positivity may have been due to metaplasia or chronic inflammation. In two of these remaining four patients a peripheral lung density was proven to be lung cancer, but the central bronchial fluorescing sites may have been due to chronic inflammation. The other two patients had many sputum specimens negative for carcinoma and none of the bronchoscopic specimens revealed tumor cells. Their true disease status is yet uncertain but they may not have lung cancer.

Overall Results

Of the first 38 patients studied to evaluate the imaging fluorescence bronchoscopy system and method, 22 were TP, 7 were TN, 9 were FP, and none were FN. In these 38 patients, 92 sites were evaluated by examination for positive and negative fluorescence and by brush and bite biopsies. There were 28 TP, 16 FP, 47 TN, and 1 FN sites. The FN site showed carcinoma in situ.

To determine the efficiency of the imaging fluorescing method, it is clear that a wider spectrum of patients will have to be studied. This must include a greater number of patients with carcinoma in situ and early or occult lung cancer and patients with other diseases. Nevertheless, a calculation of efficiency of fluorescence bronchoscopy from the data in his first report is of interest.

To *rule out* lung cancer in a given patient, a method should have a high sensitivity and therefore few false negatives. The system and methods we used indicate a sensitivity of almost 100% for both patients and sites (Table 3). Almost every bronchial cancer site will therefore be localized by its positive fluorescence for brush and bite biopsy. This fluorescence system has high accuracy for negative prediction (not lung cancer). Very few lung cances will be missed.

Table 3. Preliminary estimate of efficacy of fluorescence bronchoscopy

	Patients	Sites
Sensitivity $$\frac{TP}{(TP + FN)} =$$	$$\frac{22}{22 + 0} = 100\%$$	$$\frac{31}{31 + 1} = 97\%$$
Specificity $$\frac{TN}{(TN + FP)} =$$	$$\frac{7}{7 + 9} = 45\%$$	$$\frac{47}{47 + 16} = 75\%$$
Rule in $$\frac{TP}{(TP + FP)} =$$	$$\frac{22}{22 + 9} = 71\%$$	$$\frac{28}{28 + 16} = 64\%$$
Rule out $$\frac{TN}{(FN + TN)} =$$	$$\frac{7}{7 + 0} = 100\%$$	$$\frac{51}{51 + 1} = 98\%$$
Efficiency $$\frac{(TP + TN)}{(TP + FP + TN + FN)} =$$	$$\frac{22 + 7}{22 + 9 + 7 + 0} = 76\%$$	$$\frac{28 + 47}{28 + 16 + 47 + 1} = 82\%$$

To *rule in* lung cancer in a given patient, a method should have high specificity or few false positives. The accuracy of the system for positive prediction is about 64%−70%. Overall, efficiency was 76%−82%.

It is expected that specificity and efficiency can be improved to nearly 100% by decreasing the number of false positives. A light source is being developed that will allow quick, alternate or flip-flop switching between white light and violet light and fluorescing images will be increased by this immediate comparison. A beam-splitter will be used, one part for visualization and one for photography, so that a camera does not have to be attached and detached from the image intensifier. Both devices will save time that can be devoted to brush and bite biopsying, achieving greater accuracy with specimens obtained directly under both types of illumination.

Methods to improve retrieval of cells by brush biopsies have been instituted including use of the Saccomanno cytology tubes [28]. Finally, a team dedicated to this study consisting of a cytotechnologist, cytopathologist, and a final cytopathologist reader will enhance accurate cytopathological interpretations.

These measures are being applied to the next group of patients studied and are expected to reduce the false positive sites and patients to a low percentage and to increase specificity and efficiency to near 100%.

Discussion

The aim of this study was to evaluate the capability of a fluorescence bronchoscopy system [21] used to localize the site or sites of lung cancer in patients with sputum cytology positive for malignant cells. Our goal is to develop a method that is sensitive and accurate and will localize carcinoma in situ or small cancer plaques confined to the bronchial mucosa that are not visible on white light bronchoscopy. This potential has been demonstrated in the laboratory by visualizing the fluorescence from a solution containing only 0.01 µg/ml hematoporphyrin in an area 1.5 mm in diameter and 100 µm thick. That this potential can be achieved in patients has been demonstrated in this study in a case of occult lung cancer in a uranium miner (Fig. 6) and also by King [9].

To determine the diagnostic efficiency of fluorescence bronchoscopy, studies were initiated to determine true positive, true negative, false positive, and false negative patients and bronchial sites. This necessitated brush and bite biopsies of multiple fluorescing and nonfluorescing sites. A highly sensitive method is desired so that no site of cancer will be overlooked. The percentage of false negative sites should be low. The fluorescence bronchoscopy system meets these expectations (Table 3). Its sensitivity is nearly 100%. If a patient has lung cancer, he is highly likely to have positive fluorescence at the site or sites of cancer. If he does not show positive fluorescence, he is highly unlikely to have lung cancer (rule out). Only one of 32 positive fluorescing sites did not show lung cancer in these 22 true positive patients. This single false negative site was in the first patient with occult lung cancer we examined. White light bronchoscopy revealed two sites with subtle abnormality that showed positive fluorescence. A third, the false negative site, did not fluoresce; biopsy at this site showed carcinoma in situ, which is expected to show positive fluorescence in our experience. It is possible that this site might have shown positive fluorescence which was overlooked.

Our data indicate that patients with lung diseases other than cancer are not likely to be falsely diagnosed as having lung cancer by fluorescence bronchoscopy. Patients who did not have lung cancer according to extensive sputum cytology studies did not show positive fluorescence, as demonstrated by the seven true negative patients. All 20 sites that were brushed and biopsied in these seven patients were negative for cancer; there were no true positive, false positive, or false negative sites.

The above findings indicate that fluorescence bronchoscopy can rule out lung cancer in almost 100% of instances. There will be exceedingly few patients with sputum cytology positive for malignant cells who will not show a site of positive fluorescence in the tracheobronchial tree. There will therefore be very few patients who will have to be reexamined bronchoscopically.

There are two prerequisites for the accurate diagnosis of cancer to avoid false positive or false negative diagnoses. First, the cytopathological interpretation of carcinoma must be valid. Otherwise, the diagnosis of early cancer will either be mistaken or overlooked. Slides of sputum indicating tumor cells should be obtained and reinterpreted by a highly competent cytopathologist. Additional sputum samples should be obtained with clean, adequate sputum collections as described by Saccomanno [23] collected directly into preservative. Both deep cough and water aerosol induced sputum collections are required for accurate diagnosis. This sputum should be blended and then centrifuged and the sediment resuspended to retrieve as many tumor cells as possible. Double reading is then required.

A second prerequisite is the examination of the upper respiratory tract for cancer. In up to one-third of instances of occult malignancy, the cancer may be in the upper respiratory tract: in the larynx, pharynx, or at the base of the tongue [15]. Careful examination by direct laryngoscopy is necessary to localize the site of cancer when bronchoscopy shows no positive sites in the lower respiratory tract. Commonly, only visible lesions are anticipated for punch biopsy. Since upper respiratory tract cancer may be subtle or show no visible abnormality, brushings of various areas in the upper respiratory tract are required to localize cancer. These are taken by means of a small gauze swab for the cytopathological examination of direct smears and sediment. The pharynx, tongue, piriform sinuses, and larynx were carefully examined by both white light and fluorescence bronchoscopy in our patients with occult cancer. No cancer sites in the upper respiratory tract were identified.

The specificity of fluorescence bronchoscopy and its capability for ruling-in cancer will be increased mainly by decreasing the number of false positives. The latter are considered to be due to several factors. The first factor is inadequate retrieval of cells by brush and bite biopsies from positive fluorescing sites. In this study not only fluorescing sites but a number of nonfluorescing sites were biopsied to determine both true and false positives and negatives, which would ordinarily not be necessary in the clinical diagnostic application of fluorescence bronchoscopy. Skill had to be developed in the use of a new mode of visualization with new instruments. Sequential trials and modifications of some equipment had to be carried out and methods of photography were developed. In some patients in accomplishing these it was felt that too little time had remained for adequate brush and bite biopsying. Our goal was to achieve localization of small bronchial cancers within the time constraints of local anesthesia which at best allows about $1^1/_2$ h, rather than the several hours available under more costly general anesthesia.

Skill has now been developed so that bronchoscopy is efficiently carried out under the intensity of the fluorescent light provided by either the broad-band or the narrow-band filter. Bronchoscopic examination under fluorescent light now takes about 20 min. To make fluorescence bronchoscopic examination even more efficient and accurate a flip-flop light source is being developed to permit quick alternate switching between white light and violet light illumination. This will enhance the accuracy of recognition of positive fluorescence and will facilitate brush and bite biopsying directly under fluorescent light.

The techniques of retrieval and the yield of cells by brush biopsy also had to be improved. In addition to direct smears of brushings on frosted slides quickly fixed by immersion in 95% alcohol, the cytology tube devised by Saccomanno [24] is now being used.

Secretions and cells are dislodged from the brush upon its insertion into the cytology tube containing fixative. The sediment is smeared for cytological examination. More cells are retrieved. Smooth smears have to be made because dense areas of piled up cells or overstained areas can not be accurately evaluated cytologically and may be misinterpreted. Double reading is now carried out. All of the above factors and conditions relating to determining the status of disease (either cancer or other disease) require tight quality control for the accurate diagnosis and localization of lung cancer.

Another factor that possible contributed to the false positives is that areas of disease other than cancer may fluoresce, such as sites of acute or chronic inflammation or of metaplasia. No evidence is available in the literature to indicate whether other bronchial diseases than cancer fluoresce. Whether such sites can retain Hpd and positively fluoresce will be determined from future studies. If this should be the case, this will not diminish the value of fluorescence bronchoscopy. The nature of a disease causing positive fluorescence would in any event be established to be cancer or noncancer by brush and bite biopsies. A mistaken diagnosis of cancer will not be made. It is better that a method of localization has a low percentage of false positives than to miss even one site of cancer. Hemorrhagic areas may fluoresce but these were readily identified in our patients by their fluorescing images. The faint fluorescence of these few sites were not confused with the positive fluorescence (either localized or diffuse) of cancer sites.

It is expected that the specificity and the capability to rule in cancer by fluorescence bronchoscopy will be increased to over 90% by the measures described above to decrease false positives. Additional methods to increase specificity will be by developing instruments to measure and quantify the intensity of fluorescence. This may help to differentiate the fluorescence of bronchial cancer sites from that of diseases that may fluoresce to variable degrees, differences now not perceived or appreciated by visualization or photography.

Since Ikeda developed the fiberoptic bronchoscope, no advanced technology has been applied to extract more information from fiberoptic bronchoscopic fields or images. The analysis of images of fluorescing sites by digital computer methods will be carried out to quantify the positive fluorescence from small bronchial cancers and aid in specific diagnosis and accurate localization. The contrast between the fluorescing image and background can be enhanced and the edges of images can be better defined by digital computer methods. Analysis of the details of the topographic characteristics of fluorescing images may aid in more specifically differentiating cancer from other diseases.

Video monitor viewing at the time of fluorescence bronchoscopy will aid in making the immediate decisions required to determine whether sites are positively fluorescing or not. The video cassette tape record with concomitant voice recording will by later study enhance the accuracy of data retrieval, and will provide a permanent record for all those concerned with the diagnosis and treatment of the patient to view.

The fluorescence bronchoscopy method and system reproducibly and reliably detects bronchial cancer sites with precision (Table 2). It detects all the main histologic types of cancer. The Hpd preparation used was without toxicity, and skin photosensitivity, the only side effect to be observed, was not a significant problem. The clinical application of the fluorescence bronchoscopy method of localizing lung cancer has been shown to be practical.

Further work will now be directed toward carcinoma in situ to establish more firmly and document the capability and specificity of fluorescence bronchoscopy in localizing mucosal cancer sites that are invisible upon careful white light bronchoscopic examination.

Of clinical value will be a study to search for the extensions of cancer along a bronchus proximal from the main site, which are not visible on white light bronchoscopy but may be visualized because of their fluorescence. This will aid the thoracic surgeon in deciding the extent of lung that has to be resected so as not to leave cancer behind in the transected bronchial stump. Bronchial cancers may occur at two or more sites in one lung or in both lungs. Their efficient detection by fluorescence bronchoscopy is essential in deciding appropriate therapy.

The methods of quantitation of fluorescence to be developed together with studies of dosimetry of Hpd and light intensity will provide a basis for the localized photoradiation therapy of lung cancer. Palliative photoradiation or light therapy of large obstructing endobronchial cancers is now under way to open up blocked areas of lung for ventilation and to reduce complication from infection distal to the obstruction. The advantage of photoradiation therapy is that since Hpd is retained at higher concentration in cancer than in surrounding normal tissues, the latter are not irreversibly harmed or destroyed. The tumor selectively and preferentially absorbs light provided through the bronchoscope. Free radicals break down the cell membranes of tumor cells so they subside, while adjacent tissues are not harmed, which is not the case with the ionizing radiation of X-ray therapy.

There is a real potential of photoradiation therapy for controlling or even eradicating small bronchial cancers, as an alternative to resection. Localized photoradiation therapy will be particularly useful in patients inoperable or at high risk for surgical resection because of heart, lung, or other disease. To achieve the control or cure of bronchial cancers will require the knowledge that will result from studies of the characteristics of the fluorescent images and of the quantitation of the intensity of fluorescence at cancer sites, in order to understand dosimetry of Hpd and of light therapy. Of primary importance for the cure of early lung cancer is the sensitivity and efficiency of fluorescence bronchoscopy in localizing one or more cancer sites in the upper and lower respiratory tract.

Acknowledgements. Development of the fluorescence bronchoscope system and digital computer image analyzing instrumentation and methods is being supported by the Division of Biological Environmental Research of the United States Department of Energy, under Contract EY-76-S-03-0013 with the Medical Imaging Sciences Group. Development of clinical fluorescent bronchoscopy procedures and methods are being supported by Grant 5R01 Ca 25582 from the National Cancer Institute. Essential support is by a Grant (GCRC RR-43) from the General Clinical Research

Centers Program of the Division of Research Resources, National Institutes of Health. The Pulmonary Disease Section, Los Angeles County-USC Medical Center provided important bronchoscopic instruments, facilities and assistants essential to this research. We are grateful to Spectra Physics, Mountain View, California for the loan of the laser light source.
We gratefully acknowledge the ongoing consultation, collaboration and the providing of hematoporphyrin derivative (Hpd) by Thomas J. Dougherty, Ph.D., Head, Radiation Biology, Roswell Park Memorial Institute, Buffalo, New York. We particularly appreciate and acknowledge the close collaboration, continued encouragement and support of Geno Saccomanno, M.D., Ph.D., St. Mary's Hospital, Grand Junction, Colorado. Dr. Saccomanno referred patients with occult lung cancer who were uranium miners for fluorescence bronchoscopy. He is the final cytopathologist reader of brush and bite biopsies. He has evaluated our methods and results of sputum and brush biopsy retrieval of cells and has provided advanced training for our cytotechnologist. His extensive experience and expertise has been essential in upgrading our cytopathological methods.
Monina Labis, CT (ASCP), cytopathology technologist, worked avidly in many areas to assist in this study, including preparation of sputum and brush biopsy specimens, and in the collation of the slides and of the reports of the results on these particular patients.
Dr. C. Peter Schwinn, Head, and Dr. Timothy S. Greaves, Department of Cytopathology and cytopathology technicians afforded cytopathologic interpretation and reports for which we are grateful.

References

1. Deleted in production
2. Carden E, Phulchand PR (1975) Special new low resistance to flow tube and endotracheal tube adaptor for use during fiberoptic bronchoscopy. Ann Otol Rhinol Laryngol 84: 631−634
3. Cortese DA, Kinsey JH, Woolner LB, Payne WS, Sanderson DR, Fontana RS (1979) Clinical application of a new endoscopic technique for detection of in situ bronchial carcinoma. Mayo Clin Proc 54: 636−642
4. Delarue NC, Pearson FG, Thompson DW, Van Boxel P (1971) Sputum cytology screening for lung cancer. Geriatrics 26: 130−143
5. Doiron DR, Profio E, Vincent RG, Dougherty TJ (1979) Fluorescence bronchoscopy for detection of lung cancer. Chest 76: 27−32
6. Erozan YS, Frost JK (1977) Cytopathologic diagnosis of lung cancer. In: Straus MJ (ed) Lung cancer: clinical diagnosis and treatment. Grune & Stratton, New York, pp 95−106
7. Galen RS, Gambino SR (1975) Beyond normality. Wiley and Sons, New York
8. Gregoire HB Jr., Horger EO, Ward JL et al. (1968) Hematoporphyrin derivative fluorescence in malignant neoplasms. Ann Surg 167: 820−827
9. King G, Man G, Leriche J, Amy R, Profio AE, Doiron DR (to be published) Fluorescence bronchoscopy in the localization of bronchogenic carcinoma. Cancer
10. Kinsey JH, Cortese DA, Sanderson DR (1978) Detection of hematoporphyrin fluorescence during fiberoptic bronchoscopy to localize early bronchogenic carcinoma. Mayo Clin Proc 53: 594−600
11. Kundel HL (1979) Images, images quality and observer performance. Radiology 132: 265−271

12. Lipson RL, Baldes EJ, Olsen AM (1961) Hematoporphyrin derivative: a new aid for endoscopic detection of malignant disease. J Thorac Cardiovasc Surg 42:623–629
13. Lipson RL, Baldes EJ, Olsen AM (1964) Further evaluation of the use of hematoporphyrin derivative as a new aid in endoscopic detection of malignant disease. Dis Chest 46:676–679
14. Marsh B (1982) Bronchoscopic localization of occult lung tumors. This symposium, pp 87–89
15. Martini N, Melamed MR (1980) Occult carcinoma of the lungs. Ann Thorac Surg 30:215–223
16. Martini N, Beattie EJ, Cliffton EE, Melamed MR (1974) Radiologically occult lung cancer: report of 26 cases. Surg Clin North Am 54:811–823
17. McNeil BJ, Collins JJ Jr, Adelstein SJ (1977) Rational for seeking occult metastases in patients with bronchial carcinoma. Surg Gynecol Obstet 144:389–393
18. Mountain CF (1980) Surgical therapy of lung cancer. In: Fishman AF (ed) Pulmonary diseases and disorders. McGraw-Hill, New York, pp 1422–1429
19. Pearson FG, Thompson DW, Delarue N (1967) Experience with the cytologic detection, localization and treatment of radiologically undemonstrable bronchogenic carcinoma. J Thorac Cardiovasc Surg 54:371–382
20. Potsaid MD (1980) Diagnostic imaging in perspective. JAMA 243:2412–2417
21. Profio AE, Doiron DR, King EG (1979) Laser fluorescence bronchoscope for localization of occult lung tumors. Med Phys 6:523–525
22. Ransohoff DF, Feinstein AR (1978) Problems of spectrum and bias in evaluating the efficacy of diagnostic tests. N Engl J Med 299:926–930
23. Saccomanno G (1978) Diagnostic pulmonary cytology. Am Soc Clin Pathol, Chicago
24. Saccomanno G (1982) The contribution of uranium miners to lung cancer histogenesis. This symposium, pp 43–52
25. Saccomanno G, Archer VE, Auerbach O, Sanders RP, Brennan LM (1974) Development of carcinoma of the lung as reflected in exfoliated cells. Cancer 33:256–270
26. Sanderson DR, Fontana RS (1975) Early lung cancer detection and localization. Ann Otol Rhinol Laryngol 84:853–858
27. Sanderson DR, Fontana RS, Lipson RL, Baldes EJ (1972) Hematoporphyrin as a diagnostic tool. Cancer 30:1360–1372
28. Weinstein MD, Fineberg HW, Elstein HS, Neuhauser D, Newtra RP, McNeil BJ (1980) Clinical decision analysis. WB Saunders, Philadelphia
29. Woolner LB, Anderson HA, Bernatz PE (1960) "Occult" carcinoma of the bronchus: a study of 15 cases of in situ or early invasive bronchogenic carcinoma. Dis Chest 37:278–288
30. Woolner LB, David E, Fontana RS, Anderson HA, Bernaty PE (1970) In situ and early invasive bronchogenic carcinoma. J Thorac Cardiovasc Surg 60:275–290

Fluorescence Fiberoptic Bronchoscopy in the Diagnosis of Early Stage Lung Cancer

Y. Hayata, H. Kato, J. Ono, Y. Matsushima, N. Hayashi,
T. Saito, and N. Kawate

Tokyo Medical College, Department of Surgery, 6-7-1, Nishishinjuku, Shinjuku-ku,
Tokyo 160, Japan

Introduction

The diagnosis of early stage lung cancer developing in larger bronchi can be extremely difficult on the basis of radiological findings alone. The advent of the fiberoptic bronchoscope has improved diagnostic results but there are still cases, particularly occult cases, that present problems in localization. Increasingly widespread use of sputum cytologic examinations in surveys of high risk populations have contributed to the detection of carcinoma in situ [9] and in such cases tumor localization represents the most important subsequent step.

Recently, increasing attention has been paid to fluorescence bronchoscopy using a derivative of hematoporphyrin for localization of early lung cancer [2, 5]. The fact that hematoporphyrin accumulates in tumor tissue and emits a red fluorescence has been known for over 30 years [1, 4]. Further development in the use of this substance has been prevented by the crudeness of the material, side effects, and problems of instrumentation. In 1960, Lipson reported that hematoporphyrin derivative (Hpd), prepared from hematoporphyrin, accumulated in tumor tissue and yielded recognizable fluorescence [6]. This substance possesses extremely interesting characteristics: it is specifically retained by malignant cells, emits a red fluorescence when excited by violet light at a wavelength of 400–410 nm, and has photodynamic properties with tumoricidal effect when excited by red light [2]. The properties of Hpd, as delineated by Kinsey et al. of the Mayo Clinic [5] are shown in Table 1. The use of Hpd in

Table 1. Properties of hematoporphyrin derivative (Kinsey et al. [5])

Chemical
   Source: whole blood
   Empiric formula: $C_{34}H_{38}O_6N_4$
   Storage life: $\leq$ 1 year in saline in dark at 4° C

Biologic
   Standard dose: 2–4 mg/kg
   Uptake ratio: cancer/normal $\geq$ 10
   Persistance in tissue: 24–72 h
   Elimination pathway: liver and gastrointestinal tract

Recent Results in Cancer Research, Vol. 82
© Springer-Verlag Berlin · Heidelberg 1982

photoirradiation therapy of malignant tumors has been reported by Dougherty et al. [3].

We have used Hpd and a laser system for the photodetection of bronchogenic carcinoma first in a canine lung cancer model and subsequently in patients. This paper presents the preliminary results of this diagnostic application of Hpd.

Materials and Methods

Hematoporphyrin derivative was obtained through the courtesy of Dougherty who prepared the material by a modification of Lipson's method [3]. Profio et al. [8] have shown that when Hpd was excited by light from a mercury arc lamp with barrier filters to eliminate light of a wavelength beyond approximately 405 nm, two peaks of fluorescence at 630 nm and 690 nm were obtained. However, this system produces a background fluorescence of the same wavelength as the Hpd emitted fluorescence required for photodetection. To minimize this problem, we have used a krypton ion laser (Spectra-Physics model 164-11, wavelength: 406.7–422.6 nm, power: 1 W). An interference filter is employed to obtain a beam of light which is transmitted via a quartz fiber inserted through the instrumental channel of a BF-B3 fiberoptic bronchoscope. Fluorescence is observed via an image intensifier [2] first developed by Profio and Doiron [8]. The system is shown in Figs. 1 and 2.

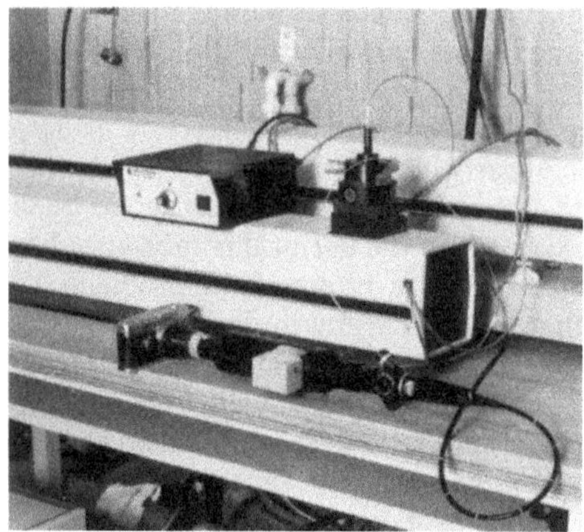

Fig. 1. Quartz fiber connected with a krypton laser and inserted through the side channel of a fiberoptic bronchoscope, to which an image intensifier and camera are attached

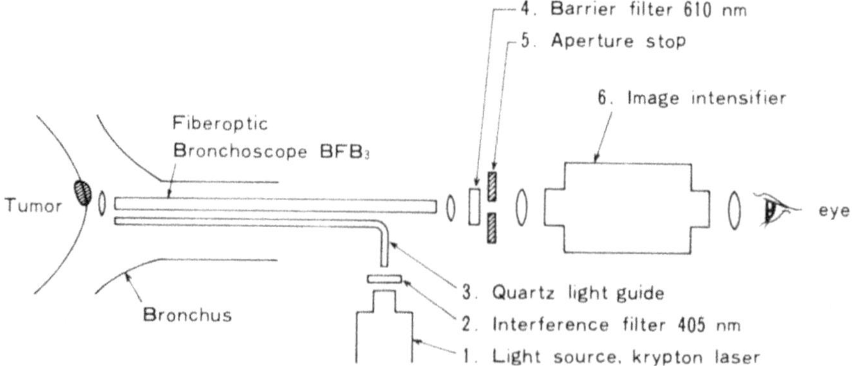

Fig. 2. Diagram of the system used for fluorescence bronchoscopy

In every case Hpd was injected intravenously 48 h before fluorescence bronchoscopy. Dosage ranged from 2.5 to 3.0 mg/kg in dogs, and from 2.5 to 4.0 mg/kg in patients.

Experimental lung cancer was induced in dogs by submucosal injection of 20-methylcholanthrene at the bifurcation of the right apical and cardiac lobe according to a method described by Kato et al. (this Symposium).

Fluorescence bronchoscopy was first performed in seven dogs with invasive squamous cell carcinoma, and in five dogs with severe atypical metaplasia. Three control dogs in which seven normal bronchial mucosa sites were selected for fluorescence broncho- scopy, were also studied. Subsequently, 16 patients with bronchogenic carcinoma, including one with an occult tumor, and one patient with severe atypical squamous metaplasia underwent fluorescence bronchoscopy. Histologic diagnosis was obtained before fluorescence bronchoscopy in all cases.

Results

Canine Lung Cancer

In six of seven dogs in which invasive squamous cell carcinoma had developed, fluorescence was recognized at the site of the tumor. In all five dogs in which severe atypical squamous metaplasia had developed, fluorescence was also recognized (Table 2). No fluorescence was observed in the normal bronchial epithelium of the

Table 2. Fluorescence of canine lung lesions using intravenous Hpd and a krypton ion laser system

Dog	Site of lesion	Pathology	Hpd dose (mg/kg)	Fluo- rescence
1. Beagle 9	Right 1st bifurcation	Sq. cell carcinoma	3.0	−
2. Beagle 12	Right 1st bifurcation	Sq. cell carcinoma	2.5	+
3. Beagle 13	Right 1st bifurcation	Sq. cell carcinoma	2.5	+
4. Beagle 16	Right 1st bifurcation	Sq. cell carcinoma	3.0	+
5. Beagle 17	Right 1st bifurcation	Sq. cell carcinoma	3.0	+
6. Beagle 21	Right 1st bifurcation	Sq. cell carcinoma	3.0	+
7. Mongrel 10	Right 1st bifurcation	Sq. cell carcinoma	2.5	+
8. Beagle 5	Right 1st bifurcation	Severe sq. metaplasia	3.0	+
9. Beagle 11	Right 1st bifurcation	Severe sq. metaplasia	2.5	+
10. Beagle 15	Right 1st bifurcation	Severe sq. metaplasia	3.0	+
11. Beagle 18	Right 1st bifurcation	Severe sq. metaplasia	3.0	+
12. Beagle 20	Right 1st bifurcation	Severe sq. metaplasia	3.0	+
1. Beagle 12	Left 1st bifurcation	Normal	2.5	−
2. Mongrel 10	Left 1st bifurcation	Normal	2.5	−
	Carina	Normal	2.5	−
3. Mongrel 17	Left 1st bifurcation	Normal	2.5	−
	Carina	Normal	2.5	−
	Right 1st bifurcation	Normal	0.5[a]	+
	Right 2nd bifurcation	Normal	2.5	−

[a] Submucosal injection

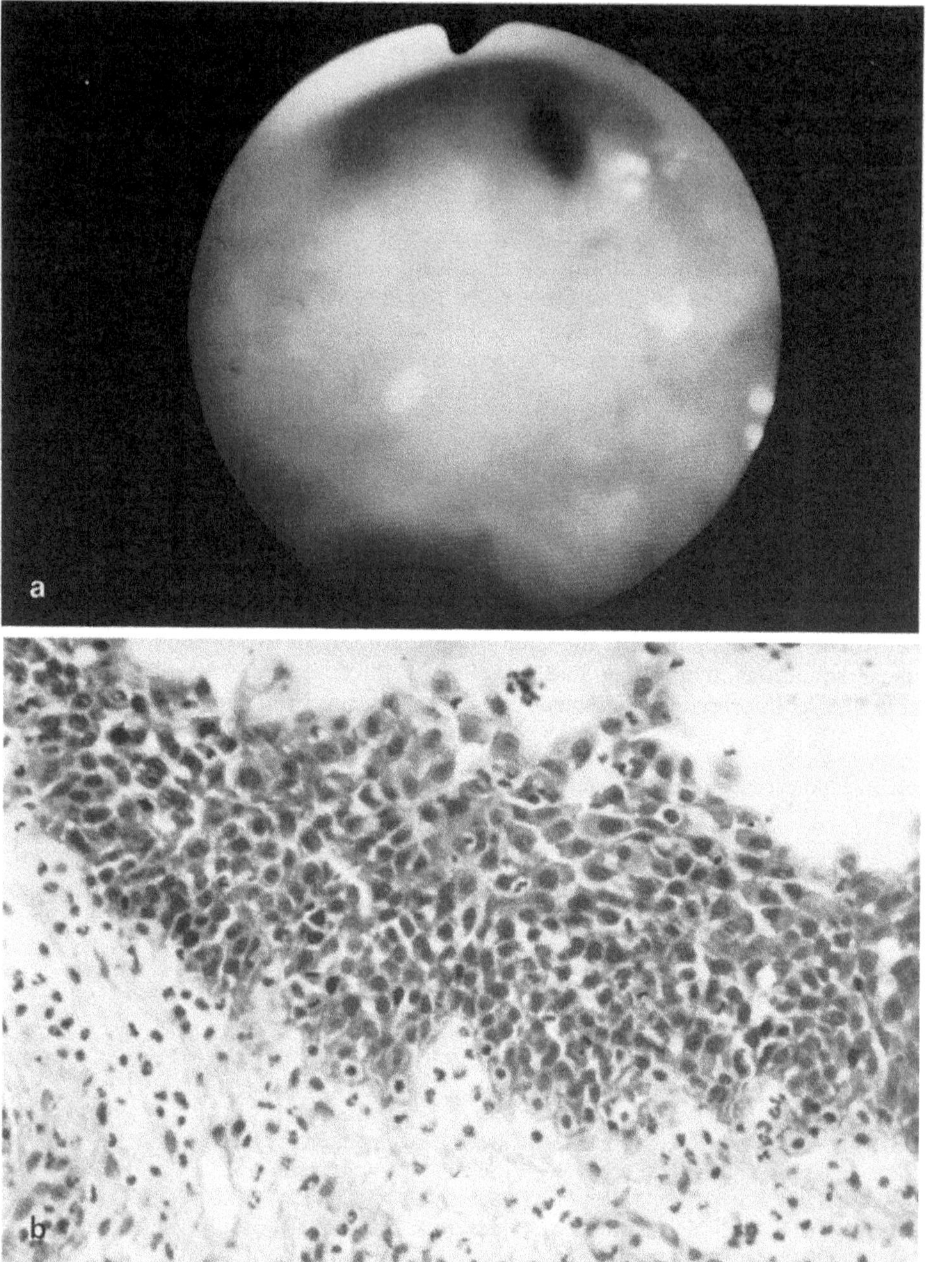

Fig. 3a–c. Canine lung cancer induced by submucosal injection of 20-methylcholanthrene. **a** White light fiberoptic bronchoscopy showing thickening and irregularity of the bronchial wall. **b** Histologic specimen showing early invasive squamous cell carcinoma. Hematoxylin-eosin × 200. **c** Fluorescence of the lesion

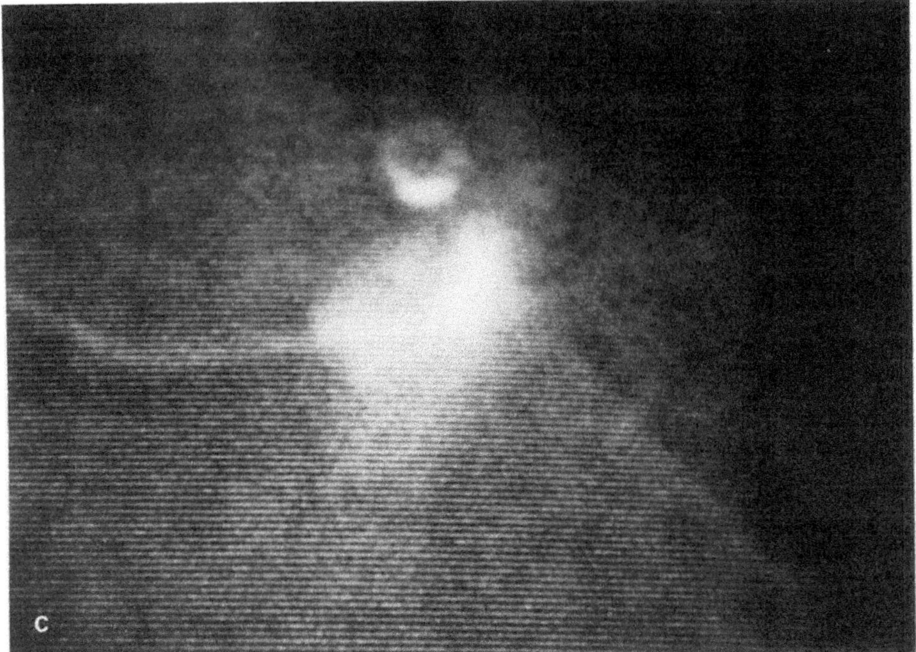

Fig. 3c. Legend see p 124

control dogs in which 2.5 mg/kg of Hpd was injected intravenously. However, fluorescence was observed at the site of a submucosal injection of 0.5 mg/kg of Hpd (Table 2). Figure 3a shows the bronchofiberscopic findings of an invasive carcinoma that developed at the bifurcation of the right apical and cardiac lobe bronchi of a dog 72 weeks after the submucosal injection of 20-methylcholanthrene; the histologic type was squamous cell carcinoma (Fig. 3b). Fluorescence bronchoscopy was performed 48 h after the intravenous injection of Hpd at a dose of 2.5 mg/kg, and fluorescence was recognized at the site of the tumor (Fig. 3c).

Human Lung Cancer

In 13 of 16 cancer cases studied 48 h after an intravenous injection of Hpd at a dose of 2.5–4.0 mg/kg, fluorescence was recognized at the site of the tumor (Table 3). Figure 4 shows the bronchofiberscopic findings in a 39-year-old woman with a large cell carcinoma located in the right upper lobe bronchus. In this case fluorescence was observed covering a wide area corresponding to that of the lesion. Figure 5 shows the bronchofiberscopic findings in a 74-year-old man with negative X-ray and positive sputum cytology. Fiberoptic bronchoscopy revealed two smoothly surfaced small tumors in the B_2 segment of the right lung. Squamous cell carcinoma was diagnosed cytologically and histologically (Fig. 6). Fluorescence was recognized coinciding with the site of the tumors.

Figure 7a shows the fiberoptic bronchoscopic findings of a 61-year-old woman in whom severely atypical squamous metaplastic cells were obtained from the site of a slight irregularity in the right upper lobe bronchus by brushing cytology (Fig. 7b): fluorescence was noted at this site (Fig. 7a).

Table 3. Fluorescence of lung lesions in patients using intravenous Hpd and a krypton ion laser system

Patient	Age	Sex	Site of lesion	Stage	Pathology	Hpd dose (mg/kg)	Fluorescence
1. T. M.	74	M	R. B_2[a]	I	SCC[c]	2.5	+
2. T. H.	56	M	R. B_9[b]	I	SCC	2.5	+
3. A. R.	60	M	R U L	II	SCC	2.5	+
4. T. T.	38	F	R U L	III	Large cell ca	2.5	+
5. M. O.	62	M	R M L	III	SCC	2.5	+
6. S. M.	50	M	$R-S_1$; R main stem	III	LCC	4.0	−[e]
7. T. S.	79	M	Lingula	III	Small cell ca	2.5	+
8. K. I.	54	M	R U L	III	SCC	2.5	+
9. M. K.	70	M	L L L	III	SCC	2.5	+
10. M. K.	61	M	L U L	III	SCC	2.5	+
11. H. U.	75	M	R main stem	IV	SCC	2.5	+
12. E. Y.	40	F	R U L	IV	Adenocarcinoma	2.5	+
13. H. Y.	65	M	R M L	IV	Small cell ca	4.0	+
14. S. K.	68	M	R. B_6	IV	SCC	2.5	−[f]
15. T. T.	71	M	R M L	IV	Large cell ca	3.0	+
16. T. M.	69	M	L U L	IV	Adenocarcinoma	2.5	−[e]
17. K. K.	61	F	R U L	0	Metaplasia[d]	2.0	+

[a] Two lesions 2 mm in diameter
[b] Lesion 1 cm in diameter
[c] Squamous cell carcinoma
[d] Severe atypical squamous metaplasia
[e] Submucosal lesion
[f] Tumor necrosis

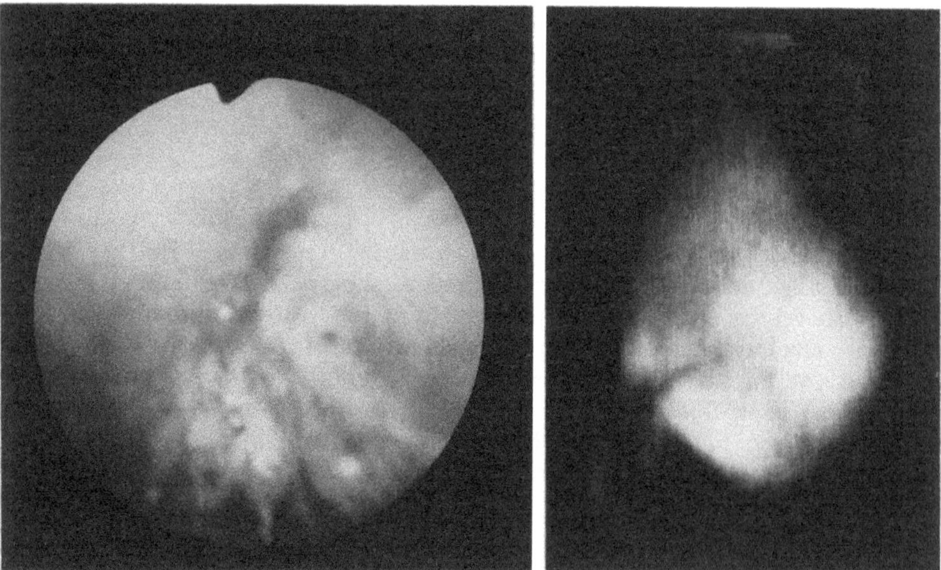

Fig. 4. Fiberoptic bronchoscopy of a 38-year-old woman under white light showing an irregular tumor obstructing the right upper lobe bronchus (*left*). Fluorescence was seen to coincide with the tumor site (*right*)

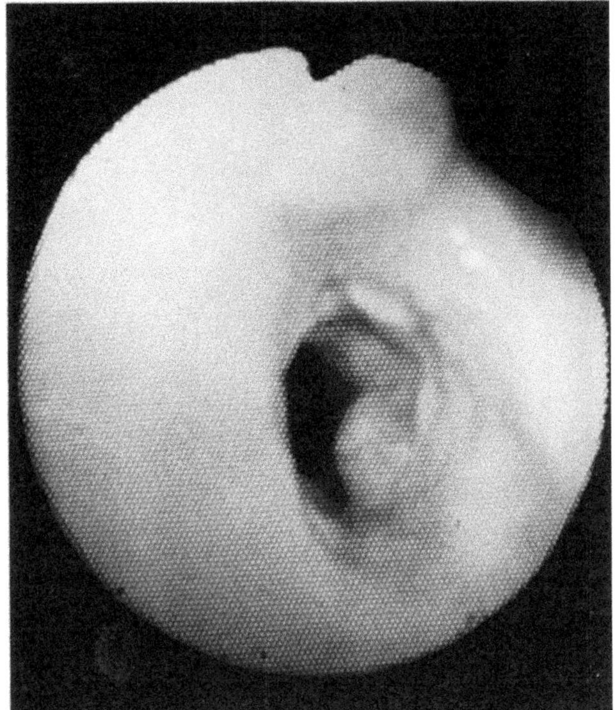

Fig. 5. Two small, smoothly surfaced tumors were recognized in the right B_2 of a 74-year-old man with negative chest X-ray and positive sputum cytology

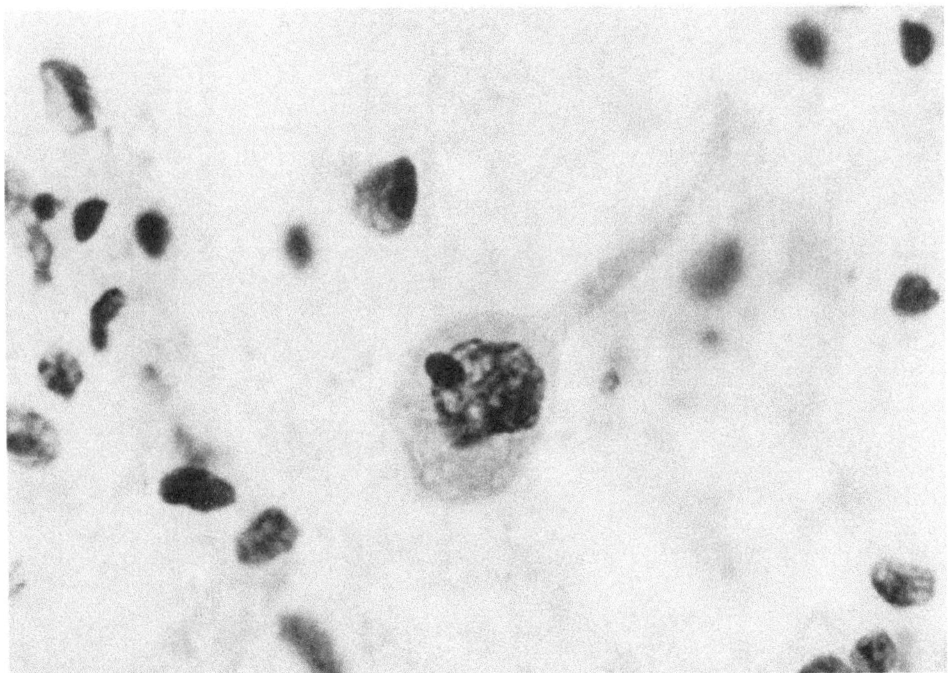

Fig. 6. Brushing cytology of the case shown in Fig. 5 revealing squamous cell carcinoma. Papanicolaou stain × 400

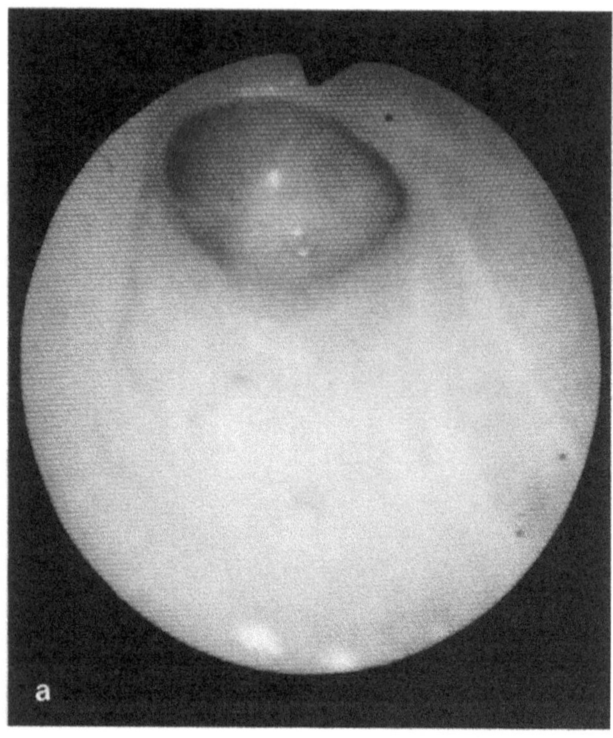

Fig. 7a, b. Legend see p 129

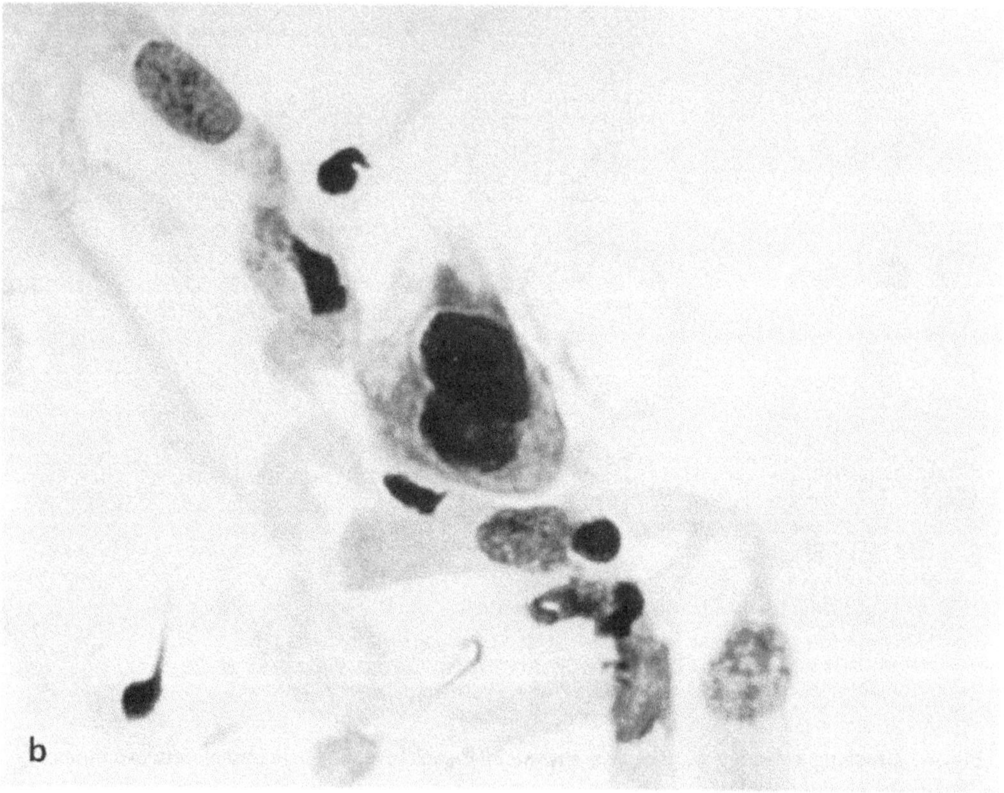

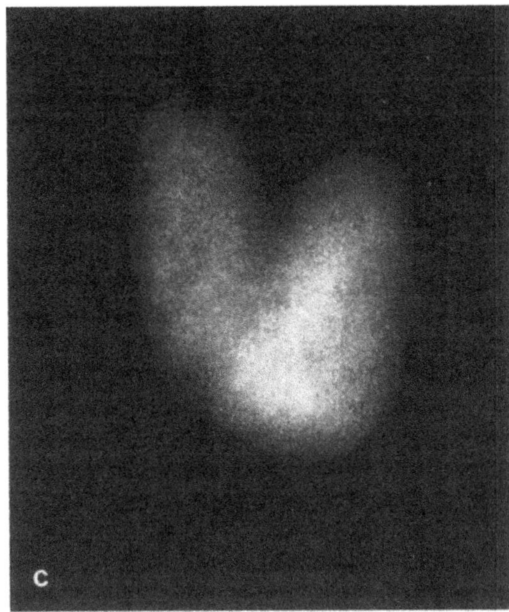

Fig. 7a–c. Squamous cell metaplasia in a 61-year-old woman. **a** Very slight irregularity in the right upper lobe bronchus seen under white light fiberoptic bronchoscopy. **b** Severe atypical squamous cell metaplasia obtained by brush cytology. **c** Faint fluorescence of the lesion

Discussion

We have performed fluorescence bronchoscopy using Hpd and a laser system in seven dogs with lung cancer, five dogs with severe squamous cell metaplasia, and in 17 patients, 16 of whom had bronchogenic carcinoma and one had severe squamous cell metaplasia of the bronchus. All four major histologic types of lung cancer fluoresced, as shown in Table 3. Fluorescence at the site of the tumor was observed in all cases except in one canine lung cancer and in three patients with bronchogenic carcinoma. The negative results can probably be ascribed to surface necrotic tissue, or to submucosal lesions (Table 3).

At a UICC workshop on "Hematoporphyrin Derivative for Detection and Treatment of Cancer" held in October 1979 in Buffalo, Cortese reported, using Hpd with a mercury arc lamp light source and an audio signal system [3], one occult lung cancer case which was not recognizable by standard white light fiberoptic bronchoscopy. Similarly, at that same meeting, Doiron et al., using a mercury arc lamp light source, reported tumor fluorescence in four cases of lung cancer, one of which had positive cytology but was negative on chest X-ray. Thus fluorescence bronchoscopy has been shown to be effective in tumor localization not only in advanced central-type lesions but also in early invasive and occult lung cancer.

The possibility of a close relationship between atypical metaplasia, carcinoma in situ and early invasive lung cancer has been described [7, 9]. In our experiments inducing central-type lung cancer in dogs, lung cancer was always preceded by increasingly atypical squamous metaplasia (Kato et al., this Symposium). Therefore we have been following cases with moderately or severely atypical squamous cell metaplasia detected by cytology surveys of certain populations at risk. As fluorescence was positive both in dogs and in patients in all cases of severe atypical squamous cell metaplasia, we feel that fluorescence bronchoscopy may hold promise in detecting this condition which was associated with the development of squamous cell carcinoma in our canine lung cancer model.

No significant side effects were noted in animals or in humans, but all patients were firmly enjoined to stay indoors after treatment because of the risk of photosensitization. No changes were noted in the normal bronchial epithelium from the laser beam.

Fluorescence bronchoscopy appears to be a safe and effective diagnostic tool to localize carcinoma of the lung and atypical squamous metaplasia.

Acknowledgments. Supported in part by a Grant-in-Aid for Scientific Research from the Ministry of Education.

The authors wish to express their deep gratitude to Dr. E. C. Holmes of U.C.L.A., Dr. T. J. Dougherty of Roswell Park Memorial Institute, Dr. P. Band of the Montreal Cancer Institute, Dr. E. G. King of the University of Alberta, Dr. D. R. Doiron and Dr. E. Profio of the University of California at Santa Barbara, and Dr. G. Huth of the University of Southern California

References

1. Auler H, Banzer G (1942) Untersuchungen über die Rolle der Porphyrine bei geschwulstkranken Menschen und Tieren. Z Krebsforsch 53:65–68
2. Doiron DR, Profio E, Vincent RG, Dougherty TJ (1979) Fluorescence bronchoscopy for detection of lung cancer. Chest 76:27–32
3. Dougherty TJ, Kaufman JE, Goldfarb A, Weishaupt KR, Boyle D, Mittleman A (1978) Photoradiation therapy for the treatment of malignant tumors. Cancer Res 38:2628–2633
4. Figge FHJ, Weiland GS, Manganiello LOJ (1948) Cancer detection and therapy: affinity of neoplastic embryonic, and traumatized tissues for porphyrins and metalloporphyrins. Proc Soc Exp Biol Med 68:640–641
5. Kinsey JH, Cortese DA, Sanderson DR (1978) Detection of hematoporphyrin fluorescence during fiberoptic bronchoscopy to localize early bronchogenic carcinoma. Mayo Clin Proc 53:594–599
6. Lipson RL, Baldes EJ (1960) The photodynamic properties of a particular hematoporphyrin derivative. Arch Dermatol 82:508–516
7. Nasiell M (1967) Abnormal columnar cell findings in bronchial epithelium. A cytologic and histologic study of lung cancer and non-lung cancer cases. Acta Cytol (Baltimore) 11:397–402
8. Profio AE, Doiron DR (1977) A feasibility study of the use of fluorescence bronchoscopy for localization of small lung tumors. Phys Med Biol 22:949–957
9. Saccomanno G, Archer VC, Auerbach O, Saunders RP, Brennan LM (1974) Development of carcinoma of the lung as reflected in exfoliated cells. Cancer 33:256–270

Results of a Lung Cancer Detection Program in an Asbestos Industry

P. Kotin and W. Paul

Johns-Manville Corporation, Denver, CO, USA

The rationale and the mechanism for sputum cytology studies in the asbestos industry are essentially the same as those for other situations where special diagnostic procedures are used for the early diagnosis of a disease. The principles involved, the techniques employed, the skills required, and the anticipated returns, as well as the inherent limitations, have a universality beyond the specific situation of the asbestos industry.

Indeed, sputum cytology programs can be analyzed from three vantage points: (1) that of public health, particularly in the regulatory sense and in the area of social responsibility; (2) that of the discipline of pathology; and (3) that of management's responsibility or obligation, as denoted by one corporation's efforts, those of Johns-Manville.

Public Health

From a public health viewpoint, sputum cytology should achieve the following goals in order to be considered a reliable and valid tool in the study of occupational disease.

Firstly, it should detect cancer cells derived from the lung at an early enough stage to permit the immediate implementation of a full diagnostic protocol so that definitive treatment can be undertaken. This goal, of course, is predicated on the assumption that early diagnosis and treatment is the major element in improving the prognosis of a patient with lung cancer.

Secondly, it should identify changes in exfoliated cells, which are potential precursors of malignant change. Such identification will allow for altering environmental exposures and for changing life-styles where indicated in order to interfere with the progression of tissue changes to cancer. It is imperative that this procedure be followed by planned monitoring and surveillance of the individual at risk so as to measure the impact of interference on the natural history of any lesion. The ultimate goal is the prevention of cancer.

Thirdly, it should serve as a biomonitor for known or suspected high-risk environments, especially in the workplace, and for identifying the presence or absence of modifying cofactors. This function will also contribute to meeting the ongoing worldwide need for data to discriminate between the environmental presence of a

Recent Results in Cancer Research, Vol. 82
© Springer-Verlag Berlin · Heidelberg 1982

potential hazard and the *actuality* of a hazard. Further, it could help in providing data to resolve such important issues as dose response, no adverse effect level and reversibility of change.

Finally, it should contribute toward the evaluation of cytologic techniques and the assessment of the usefulness of these techniques, when appropriately applied, in the control of malignant disease.

The first two goals seem straightforward enough; the second two are rather more involved.

One of the primary concerns in the public health area about the use of sputum cytology is that while it offers the possibility of diagnosing cancer prior to the appearance of X-ray changes, it is, in and of itself, essentially inadequate for the initiation of therapy. Additional diagnostic procedures are required, and depending on the situation in each individual case, these procedures could include: (1) X-rays of a type and scope more sensitive and more precise than routine chest X-rays (e.g., tomography/CAT scan); (2) visualization of the tracheobronchial tree by direct means such as bronchoscopy (e.g., fiberoptic exploration); (3) isotopic scan (parenchymal and pleural); (4) surgical invasion by bronchoscopy, with biopsy when site of lesion is identified; (5) surgical invasion by thoracotomy, with biopsy for diagnosis and lobectomy or pneumonectomy for definitive treatment. Newly emerging techniques, such as fluorescence bronchoscopy and others, still have to be evaluated prior to incorporation into a standardized approach.

Pathology

From the viewpoint of pathology, a sputum cytology program must be evaluated at the technical, the analytical, and the professional levels.

At the technical level, the protocol for and the quality of the sample collection from the patient, of the sample preparation for diagnosis, and of the actual screen of the prepared specimen are critical.

On the analytical level, the adequacy of the sample as collected and of the slide preparation must be determined by experienced cytotechnologists.

Finally, on the professional level, the quality of the diagnostic interpretation must be judged by experienced cytopathologists. Expertise is always important, but it probably is of lesser concern when changes fall clearly into any one of the categories of diagnosis. However, expertise becomes critically important when the specimen findings do not fall into the clearly unaltered category or the clearly malignant category. The consequence of underdiagnosis is self-evident, but the horror of overdiagnosis, though less potentially lethal, can create needless worry and stress.

Cytopathology is in danger of falling heir to the same debilitating ills that have occurred earlier with other laboratory diagnostic procedures which, though of real potential value, suffered from a situation in which the explosive need or demand for skilled services could not be met, and the incompetents, the opportunists, moved in to fill the void. Skill in cytopathology is crucial, and a major component of skill is experience. Two-day crash courses do not provide either technical or professional expertise. The average pathologist is not necessarily an experienced cytopathologist, except all too often by self-designation. Expertise becomes doubly crucial when a new procedure is being evaluated for its potential inclusion in regulations, both in relation to the well-being of the patient/worker and in relation to the wise use of limited resources.

Management

Industry has the obligation to use diagnostic procedures that are valid and reliable, and "diagnostic" is defined here as "leading to the identification of disease in the presence of symptoms". Industry also has the obligation to use screening procedures that are valid and reliable. "Screening" means the "identification of persons (workers) at potential high risk, through the presence of stigmata of exposure, pathophysiological or pathological abnormalities, or a work environment in which potentially hazardous agents are identified and a basis for their adverse effect can be suspected". Such identification should have a positive impact on morbidity and mortality.

As a diagnostic procedure, sputum cytology has proven to be valid and reliable as measured by prompt application of therapy and by its hoped-for beneficial impact on prognosis. Use of sputum cytology as a *screening procedure,* however, is still in the process of being validated, not in terms of the competency and authenticity of diagnosis, but rather in terms of its effectiveness in early identification of cases and its positive impact on morbidity and mortality [2].

We suspect that sputum cytology will ultimately have an application in selected situations; for example, positive benefits have been obtained in the testing of uranium miners [1]. Therefore, the existence of potentially high-risk populations in industry, such as asbestos workers, provides an excellent opportunity to continue assessing the effectiveness of sputum cytology as a screening procedure. Johns-Manville has developed such a research program, and the remainder of this paper will be devoted to the organization of the program and the results we have had to date.

Johns-Manville's Program

Our procedure was to divide our asbestos-using locations into geographic regions (a total of four) and select cytopathologists affiliated with either an academic medical center or a cytopathology research and diagnostic program to administer tests for employees in each region. Technicians from each Johns-Manville facility were trained by the regional cytopathologist to instruct employees in sputum collection techniques and to prepare and send the specimens for analysis. A standard protocol was developed during meetings involving all the regional pathologists, and the protocol provides for: (1) a standard method of sample collection and preparation; (2) a uniform method of reporting; (3) a method of data storage and epidemiological analysis (biostatistics); (4) uniform quality control; (5) uniform follow-up after cessation of exposure (i.e., workers who retire or quit or transfer to another job where there is no potentially hazardous exposure); (6) uniform criteria for preemployment sputum cytology testing; (7) determination of the effect of cytology on the prevention of lung cancer and the impact of cytological discovery (early diagnosis) on the natural history of cancer; and ultimately, (8) measurement of the impact of either reduction in smoking or cessation of smoking, and of environmental controls, on the natural history of cytological changes.

Of course, sputum cytology testing is most effective as part of a total respiratory surveillance program, and Johns-Manville offers comprehensive medical monitoring to employees at all locations, including periodic X-rays, pulmonary function testing, and complete physical examinations.

There are certain practical aspects of our experience with sputum cytology testing that merit brief elaboration:

1) An effective employee education program about the purposes and intent of cytology is imperative, because without the full cooperation of the workers, useful specimens cannot be obtained. A clear and easily understandable explanation of the potential achievements and the potential limitations of the test is also necessary. To implement the sputum cytology program within Johns-Manville, we held discussions with union representatives and employees, information was made available through the medical department at each asbestos-using facility, the nurses were thoroughly acquainted with the program and trained in appropriate techniques, and physicians explained the procedures to all employees and all levels of management at group information sessions. Education must also be continuous to maintain interest and participation in the program and to maintain quality. We believe that, in large measure, the successful implementation of testing at Johns-Manville plants was due to the thoroughness of the educational efforts.

2) One of the most difficult practical problems we faced was how to notify participants in the program of changes in sputum cytology in a way that generated no undue or unwarranted apprehension or stress. We developed eight notification categories as follows:
   a) Normal
   b) Atypia Mild − Smoker
   c) Atypia Moderate − Smoker
   d) Atypia Marked − Smoker
   e) Atypia Mild − Non-smoker
   f) Atypia Moderate − Non-smoker
   g) Atypia Marked − Non-smoker
   h) Carcinoma

If the result is normal or mild atypia, a simple letter is sent to the employee notifying him/her of the result. Because of the increased risk associated with cigarette smoking and asbestos exposure, however, the letter to smokers with mild atypia does recommend that the employee stop smoking. This same recommendation is made in all the other letters to smokers. In the other categories, notification of the results is incorporated along with a counseling session the physician holds with the employee. In addition, arrangements are made to repeat testing on a more frequent schedule and for any other tests or procedures the physician may deem advisable to determine the employee's medical status. Quarterly reports are submitted on each employee whose results have been in the moderate, marked, or suspicious of cancer category.

Johns-Manville's Results

The results of the Johns-Manville program can be seen in Tables 1 and 2. Although the program has been in effect about 3 years, not all plants started at the same time because of problems in beginning implementation. Layoffs, closing down of certain

Table 1. Sputum cytology program information

Location	Number of employees	Number participating	Total tests run
A	409	349	926
B	215	214	303
C	338	135	618
D	395	209	949
E	177	177	269
F	179	116	131
G	81	38	103
H	89	55	159
I	2,000	732	1,083
J	1,132	1,104	2,624
K	517	359	703
L	2,666	1,999	3,143
M	239	189	455
N	3	3	5
O	–	–	288
P	–	–	166
Q	–	–	73
Totals	8,440	5,679	11,998

Table 2. Cytology program results by category

Location	Total tests run	1 Unsatisfactory	2 Negative	3 Mild	4 Moderate	5 Marked	6 Carcinoma
A	926	85	534	296	9	2	0
B	303	21	188	91	3	0	0
C	618	38	337	233	7	1	2
D	949	51	579	303	15	1	0
E	269	10	156	91	11	0	1
F	131	54	60	17	0	0	0
G	103	36	60	6	1	0	0
H	159	47	98	13	1	0	0
I	1,083	236	693	148	5	0	1
J	2,624	31	2,463	127	1	0	2
K	703	13	628	60	2	0	0
L	3,143	112	2,868	155	5	2	1
M	455	38	268	140	9	0	0
N	5	0	2	2	0	0	1
O	288	11	147	122	7	1	0
P	166	24	127	14	1	0	0
Q	73	0	57	16	0	0	0
Totals	11,998	807	9,265	1,834	77	8	8

manufacturing lines and other personnel and production actions have also affected the program. However, Table 1 shows the number of locations involved in the program, the number of employees at each location at the time the program started, the number of employees participating in the program, and the total number of tests run to date. The variability in numbers of employees participating at each location can be attributed to varying union/management attitudes, location of plant (urban or rural) and the zeal and energy with which the program was introduced by management and the medical staff at the particular location.

Table 2 categorizes the test results at each location. Categories 1, 2, and 3 represent total number of tests with those results and therefore include repeats. Categories 4, 5, and 6 represent the actual number of employees having those results. It is interesting to note the differences between locations in numbers of unsatisfactory results; again, these differences result from the variations in effectiveness of management/medical staff educational and training efforts at each location. Also, it is important to note the few cases of marked atypia and carcinoma. Of the seven cases with results indicating marked atypia, five have as yet no X-ray or clinical confirmation of a neoplasm. These employees are all under special surveillance. In one case, the employee was known to have leukemia and was undergoing treatment; he subsequently died. In the remaining one case, X-rays continued to be negative but further investigation revealed an epidermoid cancer. This worker underwent a pneumonectomy and has received chemotherapy. The employee had smoked for almost 30 years. although he quit smoking about 7 years prior to sputum cytology testing. He is still alive and well since the original findings in March of 1979. What effect the early intervention will have on the prognosis in this case is still questionable.

Of the eight cases with sputum results indicating carcinoma, two cases were X-ray positive before cytology, three cases had positive X-rays immediately after cytology was found positive, and the remaining three cases have had negative X-rays both before and after cytology. In two of the cases with negative X-rays prior to cytology, the employees did have evidence of asbestosis. It may be that under certain conditions, asbestosis can mask primary X-ray changes.

In the clinical course or treatment of the carcinoma cases, five employees have had resections, with one of these having two resections. Four employees have been biopsied and there have been two laryngectomies. Five employees have received chemotherapy and one has undergone radiation treatment. Of the eight carcinoma cases, three have died since diagnosis; three are alive with continued treatment; one is undergoing further tests, and the remaining one has refused treatment.

We have had several cases in which neoplasms in employees were not picked up by sputum cytology. At one location, two employees who refused to participate in the testing program were later found to have developed malignancies. In another case, an employee's results indicated moderate atypia, but the employee did not cooperate in follow-up testing. This worker later retired and cancer was diagnosed during retirement. In the final two cases, sputum results indicated moderate atypia, but two follow-up tests in each case were negative. One neoplasm finally showed up on X-ray but was inoperable at that point. In the other case, the employee was out ill for an extended period and cancer was diagnosed during this period. In this case, too, the condition was inoperable.

Conclusions

1) Sputum cytology is still very much in the research state with respect to its usefulness as a *screening* tool.
2) There is no evidence, as yet, that early diagnosis will significantly improve prognosis.
3) Data are needed on the effect of removal of a worker from a potentially high-risk environment. Will changes regress, remain stable, or progress?
4) Cytopathologic skill of the highest level is critical during the evaluative stage. Both overdiagnosis and underdiagnosis will create enormous difficulties. Without high-level cytopathologic training, false conclusions about the ultimate utility of sputum cytology may be reached.
5) There is a definite need for federal and provincial regulations with respect to cigarette smoking in the workplace, especially in the asbestos industry. In all cases of cancer found in the Johns-Manville sputum cytology program, the employees were long-term cigarette smokers, most having smoking histories of 25 years or more.

References

1. Band P, Feldstein M, Saccomanno G, Watson L, King G (1980) Potentiation of cigarette smoking and radiation: Evidence from a sputum cytology survey among uranium miners and controls. Cancer 45: 1273–1277
2. Consensus Conference on Screening for Lung Cancer, 18–20 Sept 1978: Summary. National Cancer Program Special Communication, 19 Apr 1979. National Cancer Institute, U.S. Dept of Health, Education and Welfare

Lung Cancer Mortality in Males Screened by Chest X-ray and Cytologic Sputum Examination: A Preliminary Report

M. L. Levin, M. S. Tockman, J. K. Frost, and W. C. Ball Jr.

The Johns Hopkins Medical Institutions, Baltimore, MD, USA*

Since 1969 a study of the methodology and effect of screening for lung cancer has been carried out at the Johns Hopkins Medical Institutions under the aegis and support of the National Cancer Institute. This study was expanded in 1972 into a controlled cooperative study with the participation of the Mayo Clinic Foundation and the Sloan-Kettering Center for Cancer Research.

The Johns Hopkins Lung Project (JHLP) study population consists of men aged 45 or older, who were regular smokers of cigarettes (at least one pack per day) or, if ex-smokers, had not stopped smoking more than 1 year before entering the study. A number of sources of recruitment were used, including Baltimore City and Maryland State employees, and various other employee groups. The great majority (over 80%), however, entered the study after receiving a letter addressed to all men in the Baltimore metropolitan area who were over 44 and who had Maryland State motor vehicle driver's licenses. The letter described the study and invited participation if the recipient was not under medical care for suspected or actual lung cancer, and met the age and smoking requirements. After volunteering for the study, these men were randomized into two groups. One group (referred to as the X group) was offered annual chest X-ray examinations annually for 5 years. The other group (referred to as the XC group) was offered annual chest X-ray examinations for 5 years together with annual cytological examination of aerosol-induced sputum, followed by examination of the spontaneously produced morning sputum for three consecutive mornings. In addition, this latter group was offered cytology examination of mailed-in specimens of three consecutive morning sputum collections every 4 months. A total of 10,387 men entered the study, of whom 5,161 were assigned to the annual X-ray group and 5,226 were assigned to the X-ray plus cytology examination group.

This report will be concerned chiefly with one characteristic of the screening experience to date, i.e., comparison of the observed age-specific mortality from lung cancer with that which would be expected if the screened population was subject to the lung cancer mortality rates of two large unscreened populations of male smokers.

* Support: The Johns Hopkins Medical Institutions, Baltimore, Maryland: grant number N01-CN-45037. National Cancer Institute. The Osler-V General Clinical Research Center: grant number RR00035. Out-Patient General Clinical Research Center: grant number RR00722. Baltimore, Maryland. Division of Research Resources, Department of Health and Human Services. National Institutes of Health

These population studies are (1) the experience of the U.S. Veterans from 1954 to 1969 [6] and (2) the experience of the million volunteers studied by Hammond for the period 1959–1964 [5].

The comparison of observed and expected lung cancer mortality can be made with regard to the lung cancers identified at the first screening (prevalence) or with regard to those which occurred during approximately 4 years of subsequent screening (incidence). This preliminary report will be confined to the latter (incidence) experience.

Characteristics of Screened Population

The age distribution of the screened population differed from that of all males aged 45 years and over in Baltimore City, as recorded in the 1970 census. There were more study participants aged 45–54 (58% compared with 35%). Also, the proportion of black males was lower than that of Baltimore, probably reflecting in part the higher proportion of white males having driver's licenses (Table 1). These differences decreased the expected incidence of lung cancer which would have applied if the population age distribution were closer to that of the total male population aged 45 years and older. There is an indication also, in Table 1, that the randomization procedure was not quite adequate with respect to race, resulting in an excess of nonwhite participants (chiefly blacks) in the X group. The incidence of lung cancer is higher in blacks than whites at almost every age past 45 years (Table 2). With respect to cigarette smoking, comparison of the screened population with the 1975 National Survey of Smoking [11] indicates the former was a heavier smoking population than the general population of male cigarette smokers (race not considered; Table 3). Over one-third of the screened population was in the group whose cigarette consumption per day was 40 and over, while only 19.3% of the general population fell into a similar heavy smoking category (39.5 cigarettes per day and over). The mean cigarette consumption per day reported by the screened population was 31.

Table 1. Distribution of age and race in the JHLP and in Baltimore City

Age (years)	JHLP					Baltimore City (1970)[a]	
	XC group		X group				
	No.	%	No.	%		No.	%
45–54	3,059	58.5	3,009	58.3		50,335	38.7
55–64	1,671	32.0	1,703	33.0		41,788	32.2
65 and over	496	9.5	449	8.7		37,760	29.1
Total	5,226	100.0	5,161	100.0		129,883	100.0
Race							
White	4,556	87.2	4,401	85.3		84,510	65.1
Non-white	670	12.8	760	14.7		45,373	34.9
Total	5,226	100.0	5,161	100.0		129,883	100.0

[a] 1970 Census [10]

Table 2. Lung cancer − average annual age-specific incidence rates for males, white and black, in the 3rd National Cancer Survey, 1969−1971 [3]. Cases per 100,000

Age	White	Black
45−49	57.0	111.6
50−54	111.4	182.6
55−59	185.9	291.2
60−64	279.7	351.1
65−69	375.0	392.8
70−74	420.0	419.7

Table 3. Comparison of distribution of daily cigarette consumption between the 1975 national survey of smoking and the JHLP

1975 Survey, males [11]		JHLP study population	
Current cigarette consumption per day (midpoint of consumption category)		Current cigarette consumption per day (midpoint of consumption category)	
< 10	22.8%	10	3.5%
19.5	40.5%	20	27.4%
29.5	17.4%	30	34.3%
39.5	13.5%	40	21.3%
49.5	2.1%	50	7.8%
Other	3.7%	60+	5.0%
		Ex-smokers	0.8%
29.5 and over	36.7%	30 and over	68.4%
39.5 and over	19.3%	40 and over	34.1%

JHLP mean cigarette consumption per day 31.8

Stage of Disease

Considering resectability as an indication of stage of disease, Table 4 indicates that at first screening (prevalence) the XC group experienced over 69% resectability for cure. The X group at first screening, and both the XC and X groups, at subsequent screenings (incidence), were found resectable in 42% and 47% (Table 4).

For comparison, The Cancer Surveillance, Epidemiology and End Results (SEER) program of the Division of Cancer Cause and Prevention, National Cancer Institute, has reported that in 1970−1973, 18% of white male patients with lung cancer referred to the institutions represented by the SEER program were classified as "localized" (tumor confined to the site of origin) [8]. Seventeen percent of black male patients with lung cancer were classified as localized. It is pertinent to note that during the same period (1970−1973), 19% of the white lung cancer patients were treated by surgery only; the corresponding proportion of black patients was 15% (not sex-differentiated).

Table 4. Lung cancer screening (JHLP) − resectability

		Resectability	
Prevalence	Screenee[a]	25/36	69.4%
	Control[b]	17/40	42.5%
Incidence	Screenee[a]	47/100	47.0%
	Control[b]	45/102	44.1%

[a] Screenee refers to the group screened by cytology as well as X-ray examination (XC group)

[b] Control refers to the group screened by chest X-ray only (X group)

Therefore, the resectability in the JHLP is more than twice the unselected clinical resectability reported by SEER. On the other hand, resectability in the screened JHLP population is similar to that in 450 consecutive lung cancer admissions to the surgical service of Dr. N. C. Delarue over the decade 1966−1976 at the Toronto General Hospital. This surgical series was found to have 43.5% resectability [4]. Which of the rates of clinical resectability of lung cancer (SEER or the Toronto experience) most closely approximates that of an "unscreened" population is not evident. Perhaps some proportion between 18% and 40% more closely reflects the resectability of lung cancer in the community.

Incidence

As would be expected in a smoking population, the annual incidence (new cases per year) of lung cancer in the two screened groups was high (4.6−4.9 per 1,000 person-years). The incidence among the screened smokers was more than three times that among white males in the 3rd National Cancer Survey [3] of 1969−1971 (Table 5). Since the latter survey did not distinguish between smokers and others, however, this ratio is not indicative of the excess incidence of lung cancer among cigarette smokers compared with that of nonsmokers.

Lung Cancer Mortality

The lung cancer mortality of incidence cases detected from among the XC and X groups through 30 September 1980 is given in Table 6. There was no significant difference in lung cancer mortality between the two screened groups during the approximately 4 years of observation to date.

Some earlier comparisons suggested a difference in mortality from squamous cell cancer compared to other cell types in X and XC groups. In Table 7 this comparison is shown, with our most recent data.

Mortality Compared to Population Studies

The two population studies selected for comparing lung cancer mortality with that thus far observed in our screened population included, as previous stated, that of the

Table 5. Incidence of lung cancer: Age-specific incidence rates

Age	XC group[a]			X group [b]			3rd National cancer survey (white males)
	P/years[c]	Cases per 1,000	Rate	P/years[c]	Cases per 1,000	Rate	
45−49	3,693	3	0.8	3,451	3	0.9	0.6
50−54	6,410	13	2.0	6,190	14	2.3	1.1
55−59	4,998	25	5.0	5,028	22	4.4	1.9
60−64	3,394	20	5.9	3,418	24	7.0	2.8
65−69	2,015	24	11.9	1,718	26	15.1	3.8
70+	1,022	15	14.7	842	13	15.4	4.2[d]
Total	21,532	100	4.6	20,647	102	4.9	1.5[e]

[a] Screened by X-ray and cytology (all races)
[b] Screened by X-ray only (all races)
[c] Person-years observation from entering study to diagnosis, or last observation, as of 30 September 1980
[d] Age 70−74
[e] Age-adjusted to total screenee and control population

Table 6. Lung cancer mortality in screened groups

Screened group	P/years	Lung cancer deaths	Deaths per 1,000
X-ray and cytology	21,713	51	2.35
X-ray	20,818	59 $p = 0.32$	2.83

Comparison of age-specific death-rates resulted in no significant difference: $p = 0.37$

Table 7. Incidence lung cancer mortality in the XC and X groups

Group	P/years	Deaths	Rate per 100,000
Squamous cell			
XC	21,712	8	37
X	20,818	12	58 ($p = 0.32$)
Comparison of age specific rates, $p = 0.25$			
Other cell types			
XC	21,712	43	198
X	20,818	47	226 ($p = 0.55$)
Comparison of age-specific rates, $p > 0.35$			

Table 8. Incidence of lung cancer mortality observed in a screened population and expected on basis of Veterans study, 1954–1969 [6]

XC group				X group			
Age	P/years[a]	Lung cancer deaths		P/years[a]	Lung cancer deaths		
		Expected	Observed			Expected	Observed
45–54	10,144	6.72	7	9,669	6.40	10	
55–64	8,474	17.46	17	8,528	17.51	21	
65–74	3,095	12.38	27	2,621	10.31	28	
Total	21,713	36.56	51	20,818	34.22	59	

$$\frac{\text{Obs.}}{\text{Exp.}} = 1.39$$

95% confidence limits 1.09–1.69

$$\frac{\text{Obs.}}{\text{Exp.}} = 1.72$$

95% confidence limits 1.28–2.18

[a] Person-years from entering study to death or last observation

Table 9. Incidence of lung cancer mortality observed in a screened population and expected on basis of American Cancer Society Study [5]

XC group				X group			
Age	P/years[a]	Lung cancer deaths		P/years[a]	Lung cancer deaths		
		Expected[b]	Observed			Expected[b]	Observed
45–54[a]	10,144	4.51	7	9,669	4.30	10	
55–69	10,525	32.67	30	10,279	31.91	38	
70 and over	1,044	5.02	14	870	4.18	11	
Total	21,713	42.20	51	20,818	40.39	59	

$$\frac{\text{Obs.}}{\text{Exp.}} = 1.21$$

95% confidence limits 0.88–1.54

$$\frac{\text{Obs.}}{\text{Exp.}} = 1.46$$

95% confidence limits 1.09–1.83

[a] Based on mortality at ages 35–54

290,000 U.S. life policy holders (chiefly U.S. Veterans) studied prospectively from 1 January 1954 to 31 December 1969 by Dorn and Kahn [6] and by Rogot and Murray [9]. Rogot and Murray have pointed out that in this experience of almost four million person-years extending over a 16-year period the mortality ratio from lung cancer (current smokers versus nonsmokers) was 10.9 during the first $8^1/_2$ years and 11.3 during the total 16 years, indicating no significant change in the lung cancer mortality among smokers compared with nonsmokers over the entire period.

The age-specific mortality rates in the Veterans study as reported by Kahn [6, 8] in the period 1954–1962 (the age-specific mortality rates in both the Veterans study and Hammond's study have been adjusted to the amount smoked per day distribution of the screened population) are compared to the age-specific rates among the XC and X groups in Table 8. It will be noted that there were more deaths observed than expected in each group. The 95% confidence limits for the ratio of observed to expected deaths were 1.09—1.69 in the XC group; the corresponding limits for the X group were 1.23—2.18.

Utilizing the American Cancer Society Prospective Study [10] of one million volunteers over a 4-year period, a similar comparison is shown in Table 9. The results are similar to those found with the U.S. Veterans experience. The ratio of observed to expected deaths in the XC group was not significantly different from unity; in the X group, there were more deaths observed than expected.

Comment. This study does not offer historical population studies as suitable controls for current studies, but examines a hypothesis which makes historical data appropriate. Rogot and Murray [9] have reported that lung cancer mortality in U.S. Veterans who were cigarette smokers did not change appreciably over time (1954—1969) for smokers of the same amount and age, i.e., in this large population, for given age and smoking, lung cancer mortality has remained constant. This suggested the hypothesis that given age and amount smoked, lung cancer mortality remains constant in various general populations, and is not significantly altered by a screening program. In this paper, two tests of the hypothesis were made, that from the Veterans' experience and that from E. C. Hammond's study of one million persons. Both comparisons indicated no significant difference from the lung cancer mortality of the XC group; there was some indication of excess mortality in the X group. There was no evidence of decreased mortality in either group as a result of screening. We consider these observations pertinent, although not definitive, to the evaluation of the effect of screening as well as to the general epidemiology of lung cancer.

Discussion

Among the three cooperative groups in this screening study, only one (Mayo Clinic) included a randomized *unscreened* group in the incidence series. The mortality from lung cancer in this group, when available, will constitute a third control group (in addition to the two population studies noted earlier) to compare observed lung cancer deaths in the JHLP screened population with those expected to occur from the experience of an unscreened male population of the same age and smoking status. (A preliminary examination of the Mayo control data indicates results similar to those found with the population studies.) When the presented data are compared to population studies (and possibly to a current unscreened control), the JHLP lung cancer mortality experience demonstrates no evidence of reduction in lung cancer mortality as a result of early diagnosis by X-ray and cytology screening and prompt appropriate treatment at a medical center well equipped for the diagnosis and treatment of this disease.

The absence of evidence that mass screening for lung cancer reduces lung cancer mortality in the screened population has been noted in past studies and reviews [1, 2, 7]. In general, the expectation that screening for disease would reduce mortality rests on at least two assumptions. First, that the screening process can identify a significant proportion of patients in whom the disease is at a stage less advanced ("early") in its natural history or clinical course than is usually true of clinical cases, i.e., cases diagnosed as a result of patients voluntarily seeking medical care because of symptoms. Given the first assumption, the efficacy of screening then rests on the assumption that treatment of the disease at these earlier stages results in decreased mortality in comparison with that expected in a comparable population in which the diagnosis and treatment of the disease was not preceded by the mass screening procedure. Failure of a given screening program to reduce mortality may thus be due to failure of the screening procedure to comply with either of these assumptions or with both. There is little doubt that present-day screening procedures identify a higher population of resectable cases than is usual in clinical cases, and particularly than was true at the time covered by the population studies. The question then arises: Is this increase in the proportion of early cases sufficiently large to result in an appreciable reduction of lung cancer mortality? Or is the natural history of lung cancer such that present-day treatment (chiefly surgical) may not be expected to increase the average survival of patients, age and stage of disease taken into consideration?

These observations from the continuing JHLP screening study provide no clear evidence that mass screening reduces mortality due to lung cancer. Although "early" cases have been detected, it is possible that the presently available therapies for lung cancer are not yet effective even in such early stages. There remains the possibility that some lung cancers are very slowly progressing tumors, taking as much as 10 years to become clinically apparent. Such slowly growing lung cancers may remain permanently cured if detected and removed at their earliest detectable stage. These cases would not contribute to a decrease in mortality in this study, which covers a period of less than 5 years. The multifocal nature of pulmonary neoplasms and the cardiovascular damage from cigarette smoking constitute the chief obstacles to this more hopeful aspect of the possible efficacy of lung cancer screening.

The excess of observed over expected lung cancer deaths, based on the population studies, is not readily explainable. The screened population, composed of volunteers, may contain a greater proportion of persons at risk of developing lung cancer than would be true of a more representative population of male cigarette smokers. A more precise evaluation of the observed compared with the expected lung cancer mortality may be obtained when the age-specific lung cancer mortality of the unscreened control group studied in the Mayo Clinic study is available.

Summary

Observations from the continuing JHLP lung cancer screening study provide no clear evidence that mass screening by chest X-ray and sputum cytology, plus prompt appropriate treatment, reduces mortality du to lung cancer. No reduction in lung cancer deaths is observed in the JHLP when compared with the number of lung cancer deaths expected from the experience of two unscreened male populations of the same age and smoking status serving as population studies. Possible reasons for the lack of demonstrable decrease in mortality, even though "early" cases have been detected, include: (1) an insufficient passage of time for slowly growing cancers to become apparent in the control group, (2) ineffective therapy, and (3) the multifocal nature of pulmonary neoplasms. Additional study will be required to provide a definitive answer regarding the benefit, if any, of lung cancer screening.

References

1. Boucot KR, Weiss W (1973) Is curable lung cancer detected by semi-annual screening? JAMA 224: 1361–1365
2. Brett GZ (1969) Earlier diagnosis and survival of lung cancer. Br Med J 4: 260–262
3. Cutler SJ, Young TL (eds) (1975) Third national cancer survey: incidence data. Natl Cancer Inst, Bethesda, p 118, 130
4. Delarue NC (1980) Lung Cancer in historical perspective. Can J Surg 23: 549–557
5. Hammond EC (1966) Smoking in relation to the death rates of one million men and women. In: Haenszel W (ed) Epidemiological study of cancer and other chronic diseases. Natl Cancer Inst, Bethesda, p 152
6. Kahn HA (1966) The Dorn study of smoking mortality among US veterans. In: Haenszel W (ed) Epidemiological approaches to the study of cancer and other diseases. Natl Cancer Inst, Bethesda, pp 1–125
7. Lilienfeld A, Archer PG, Burnett CH et al. (1966) An evaluation of radiographic and cytologic screening for the early detection of lung cancer. A Cooperative Pilot Study of the American Cancer Society and the Veterans Administration. Cancer Res 24: 2083–2121
8. National Cancer Institute (End Results Section, Biometry Branch, Division of Cancer Cause and Prevention) (1976) Cancer patient survival, report no. 5. Natl. Cancer Inst, Bethesda
9. Rogot E, Murray JL (1980) Smoking and causes of death among US veterans. 16 years of observation. Public Health Rep 95: 213–222
10. United States Bureau of Census and Population (1970, 1971) Census of population: general population characteristics. US Government Printing Office, Washington, DC
11. United States Department of Health, Education and Welfare. Public Health Service. National Clearinghouse for Smoking and Health (1975) Adult Use of Tobacco

Sputum Cytology and Asbestos Exposure: A Preliminary Report*

A. Simard, R. Vauclair, M. Feldstein, F. Bergeron,
N. Morissette, and P. Band

Institut du Cancer de Montréal, Hôpital Notre-Dame et Université de Montréal,
Montréal, Québec, Canada**

Introduction

The increased frequency of pulmonary cancer in uranium miners is well established
and has been attributed to the irradiation of the tracheobronchial epithelium by alpha
radiation [1].
The relationship between cigarette smoking and pulmonary cancer is well known [3,
4], and the frequency of this disease amongst uranium miners is particularly observed
in heavy smokers [2].
Sputum cytology studies of uranium miners by Saccomanno et al. [9, 10] revealed the
progression over time of atypical cellular changes preceding the development of in situ
and invasive carcinoma. Thus, cytologic detection of pulmonary cancer may antedate
by several years radiologic evidence of the tumor. In a recent sputum cytology study
among uranium miners and controls, Band et al. [2] further showed that:

1) In the absence of either risk factor (smoking or exposure to radon), the frequency
   of abnormal cytology was about 5%.
2) In the presence of one risk factor, either smoking without exposure to radon, or
   radon exposure without smoking, the frequency of abnormal cytology was
   about 10%.
3) The presence of both risk factors caused a linear increase in the frequency of
   sputum cytology abnormalities.

Based on these findings, we have undertaken the following sputum cytology study
among asbestos workers.

The Asbestos Industry

Epidemiological studies carried out over the past few decades have clearly shown that
a problem of pulmonary cancer indeed exists in asbestos mines.

* Supported by the Institute of Occupational and Environmental Health, Quebec Asbestos
 Mining Association, and by the Ministère des Affaires Sociales du Québec
** We wish to thank Mr. Willie Coulter for his programming assistance and Miss Line Bernier
 for the typing of the manuscript. The authors are also greatly indebted to Dr. Richard
 Lambert, Head of the Industrial Clinic of Thetford-Mines, and to many union and company
 representatives for their help and cooperation

Extensive surveys have confirmed that for Quebec miners and millers exposed to 400–800 MPCF-years (millions of particles per cubic foot of air × number of years of exposure), the risk of developing a respiratory cancer was 2.1. This risk increased to 3.6 for those exposed to more than 800 MPCF-years [8].
Exposures to these very high asbestos concentrations are no longer present. However, the pulmonary carcinogenic potential of low doses of asbestos remains unknown [11].

Methods

This sputum cytology study began in September 1979 and was carried out in three different asbestos companies, referred to as A, B, and C, located in the same mining community in Quebec. At the closing date of September 19, 1979, all male and female

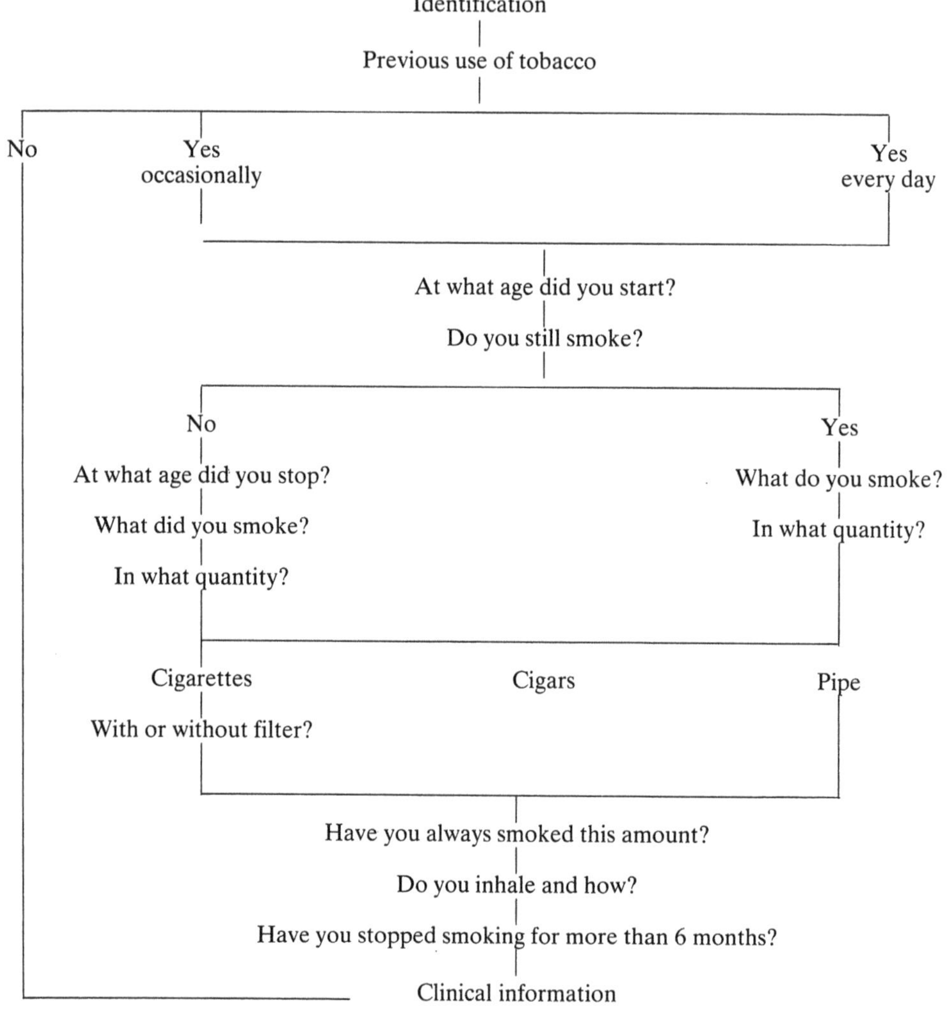

Fig. 1. Summary of the principal questions used to determine smoking history

asbestos workers with $4^1/_2$ years of exposure in mine B, and all male workers with at least 25 years of exposure in mine A were selected. Male workers in mine C who had at least 25 years of exposure at the closure date of October 10, 1980 were also selected. Although other workers who did not satisfy the above criteria were screened if they so desired, their results are not included in the present analysis.

All eligible workers were sent a letter defining the aims of the project and inviting them to participate on a voluntary basis. Those who chose to participate were interviewed individually by a member of our team in mines B and C, while workers in mine A were interviewed by the security supervisors, specifically instructed by one of us, in the three different mines and mills of that company. During the interview each participant was verbally instructed how to produce a satisfactory sputum specimen and was given a written reminder along with the bottle of fixative. The interviews were either conducted on company time or according to other schedules. All eligible workers were asked to fill in an identification questionnaire indicating their name, age, sex, and smoking status as well as past and present occupations. The questionnaire was formulated to permit the generation of a code sheet for computer entry.

Smoking history was established based upon questions indicated in Fig. 1. Workers were asked if they smoked regularly, in what amount, at which age they started smoking and about their current smoking status. The inhalation process and quantity of cigarette smoking were clearly defined. Periods of nonsmoking were only considered if they exceeded 6 months.

Exposure to asbestos will be determined by dose (low: less than 2 fibers/cm^3, medium: $2-10$ fibers/cm^3, and high: more than 10 fibers/cm^3), and by *duration* of exposure (short: less than 10 years, medium: $10-20$ years, and long: more than 20 years). Workers will also be classified according to interval from first exposure to time of sputum cytology result. Correlation between asbestos exposure and sputum cytology findings is currently in process and is not included in this report.

Sputum Cytology

Each worker received on bottle of liquid fixative (50% ethyl alcohol and 2% carbowax). Expectorations, pooled from three consecutive mornings' deep cough specimens, were sent to our laboratory. Smears processed according to the Saccomanno technique [9] were first screened by a cytotechnologist and all abnormal smears were subsequently examined by the same pathologist (R.V.).

The following criteria were used to classify cytological specimens:
1) Unsatisfactory: mostly salivary specimens
2) Negative: cellular morphology within normal limits
3) Mild atypical metaplasia
4) Moderate atypical metaplasia
5) Marked atypical metaplasia
6) Inconclusive: malignancy suspected
7) Epidermoid in situ carcinoma probable
8) Invasive epidermoid carcinoma
9) Other types of carcinomas

Specimens were judged as satisfactory using Koss's criterion [6], namely the presence of alveolar macrophages (1 per 100 × field); unsatisfactory specimens warranted a repeat without aerosol. A positive result of atypia, particularly categories 4–8, called for a repeat specimen every 3–4 months.

Results and Discussion

To date, worker participation in the screening program has generally been good, as shown in Table 1.

The preliminary results of the program, as of October 1980, are shown in Table 2. Analysis of the results from mine B have been completed, whereas nearly half of the workers from mine A are still under study. Individual smears taken from mine C employees remain to be examined.

The high percentage of unsatisfactory results obtained is due to our adherence to Koss's criterion which states that a satisfactory sputum specimen should contain an average of at least 1 alveolar macrophage per 100 × field. We feel that this criterion increases the method's reliability in detecting cells which exfoliate from minimal sized lesions of the bronchial epithelium. The mere presence of cylindrical or ciliated cells does not constitute, per se, an *acceptable criterion* since these cells may originate from the upper respiratory tract. Moreover, we have repeatedly observed in salivary specimens the presence of small immature squamous cells indistinguishable from squamous metaplastic cells of the bronchial mucosa which, occasionally, presented atypical features.

The level of participation of mine B workers who, having obtained unsatisfactory results, were sent a second bottle of fixative dropped to 36%. Of these specimens, 40 resulted in unsatisfactory smears, 57% showed normal cells, and 3% showed mild atypia.

Table 3 shows the cytological results relative to the age distribution of the workers in mine B. It should be noted that four of the six mild atypias were found in workers 40–60 years of age. Cigarette smoking has been investigated, and a preliminary classification of smoking status of mine B is given in Table 4.

From the results of our preliminary study, there is no indication of any significant increase in the rate of neoplastic or dysplastic lesions in smoking asbestos workers. We stress the point that the study must be completed in order to draw any definite conclusions. It must be kept in mind, however, that amongst smokers, the predominant pathology of lung cancer is the squamous cell type, whereas asbestos exposure is predominantly associated with the adenocarcinoma type [5, 7]. Although much data has been published in recent years concerning the pathogenesis of pulmonary epidermoid carcinoma (the progression of atypias to carcinoma in situ and to invasive carcinoma) no such data is available pertaining to the pathogenesis of lung adenocarcinomas. This is probably due to the fact that adenocarcinomas, particularly the early lesions, tend to be located in the periphery of the lung and thus do not lend themselves well to cytological detection. It is interesting to note that in those lung diseases in which pulmonary fibrosis is found, such as asbestosis, adenocarcinomas represent the most common type of malignancy encountered.

The preliminary results shown in this report concord with the findings presented by Drs. Kotin and Paul at this Symposium. These authors observed a low number of atypias and cancers in a different asbestos mine, also located in Quebec; it must also be pointed out that a high percentage of unsatisfactory specimens was noted by at least one of the pathologists participating in that study.

Table 1. Workers participation in the program

Mine	Number of workers eligible	Number of workers participating	%
A	728	579	80
B	410	225	55
C	82	68	83
Total	1,220	872	73

Table 2. Preliminary sputum cytology results

Sputum cytology	Mine A[a]		Mine B	
	No.	%	No.	%
Unreturned bottles	–	–	25	9.8
Unsatisfactory	55	18.5	65	25.6
Normal	223	74.8	158	62.2
Mild metaplasia	16	5.4	6	2.4
Moderate metaplasia	4	1.3	0	0.0
Total	298	100	254	100

[a] Incomplete results: 298 individuals examined out of a possible maximum of 579

Table 3. Sputum cytology results by age groups of workers

Cytology	Age distribution (years)					Total
	19–29	30–39	40–49	50–59	60–64	
Unreturned bottles	6	13	3	3	0	25
Unsatisfactory	15	23	14	9	4	65
Normal	17	30	43	55	13	158
Mild metaplasia	0	2	2	2	0	6
Total	38	68	62	69	17	254

Table 4. Sputum cytology distribution by smoking status of workers

Cytology	Smokers	Nonsmokers	Ex-smokers
Unreturned bottles	11 (4.3)[a]	9 (3.5)	5 (2.0)
Unsatisfactory	16 (6.3)	29 (11.4)	20 (7.9)
Normal	99 (39.0)	19 (7.5)	40 (15.7)
Mild metaplasia	3 (1.2)	1 (0.4)	2 (0.8)
Total	129 (50.8)	58 (22.8)	67 (26.4)

[a] Percentages shown in brackets

References

1. Archer VE, Wagoner JK (1973) Lung cancer among uranium miners in the United States. Health Phys 25: 351–371
2. Band P, Feldstein M, Saccomanno G, Watson L, King G (1980) Potentiation of cigarette smoking and radiation. Evidence from a sputum cytology survey among uranium miners and controls. Cancer 45: 1273–1277
3. Doll R (1978) An epidemiologic perspective of the biology of cancer. Cancer Res 38: 3573–3583
4. Doll R, Peto R (1978) Lung cancer in regular cigarette smokers: dose and time relationship in British doctors. J Epidemiol Comm Health 32: 303–313
5. Kannerstein M, Chug J (1972) Pathology of carcinoma of the lung associated with asbestos exposure. Cancer 30: 14–21
6. Koss LG (1979) Diagnostic cytology and its histopathologic bases, 3rd edn, vol 2. Lippincott
7. Preger L (1978) Asbestos related disease. Grune & Stratton, New York
8. Rohl AN, Langer AM, Selikoff IJ (1978) Chrysotile asbestos: effects of human exposure. Science 198: 1202
9. Saccomanno G, Archer VE, Auerbach O, Saunders RP, Brennan LM (1974) Development of carcinoma of the lung as reflected in exfoliated cells. Cancer 33: 256–270
10. Saccomanno G, Archer VE, Saunders RP, Auerbach O, Klein MG (1976) Early indices of cancer risk among uranium miners with reference to modifying factors. In: Saffiotti U, Wagoner JK (eds) Occupational carcinogenesis. Ann NY Acad Sci 271: 377–383
11. Selikoff IJ, Lee KHK (1978) Asbestos and disease. Academic Press, New York

Lung Cancer Screening Programs in Canadian Uranium Mines*

P. Band, M. Feldstein, L. Watson, G. King, and G. Saccomanno

Institut du Cancer de Montréal, Hôpital Notre-Dame, Montréal, Québec, Canada

Introduction

The increased incidence of lung cancer first observed among uranium miners in Europe [5], has been confirmed by epidemiologic studies in the uranium mines of the Colorado Plateau [1, 14]. This excess in lung cancer is attributed to the irradiation of the tracheobronchial epithelium by alpha particles emitted during the radioactive decay of radon gas into its short-lived radon daughters [6]. The relationship between cigarette smoking and lung cancer is well documented [15], and evidence that cigarette smoking by uranium miners is a factor in the development of lung cancer has been reported [2].
Saccomanno et al. [10, 11], in sputum cytology studies of uranium workers, have documented in individuals developing bronchogenic carcinoma, a general pattern of cellular changes consisting of atypical metaplasia becoming gradually more severe with time and ultimately progressing to carcinoma in situ and to invasive carcinoma.
Based on these premises, we have initiated a program for the early detection of lung cancer in Canadian uranium mines.

Materials and Methods

Uranium City Project

In September of 1974, a prospective survey consisting of periodic sputum cytology and chest X-ray studies was initiated in Uranium City, a uranium mining town of Northern Saskatchewan. Individuals were invited to participate on a voluntary basis and 80% of the uranium workers joined the program.

Data Collection and Procedure. Detailed health, occupational, and smoking histories were obtained by personally interviewing all participants. A standard size postero-anterior roentgenogram of the chest, and expectorations pooled from three

---

* Supported in part by the Government of Saskatchewan and Eldorado Nuclear Limited (Uranium City Project), and the Elliot Lake Centre

consecutive mornings deep cough specimens were obtained once yearly in all participants.

Sputum specimens, collected in plastic jars containing 50% ethyl alcohol and 2% Carbowax as fixatives were evaluated by one of us (G.S.) according to a classification previously described [10]. Specimens showing normal or mildly atypical cells were considered normal; those showing moderate atypia, marked atypia, or cancer cells were classified as abnormal. Sputum cytology was repeated twice yearly in individuals with moderate atypia, and three times yearly in those with marked atypia. Individuals with marked atypia underwent selective segmental fiberoptic bronchoscopy and chest X-ray studies at 4-month intervals.

A uranium miner was defined as a worker with at least 1 month of underground uranium mining experience. Individuals were classified as nonsmokers if they never smoked. The cigarette index, defined as the average number of cigarettes smoked per day multiplied by the number of years of regular smoking, was used to assess smoking history. Cumulative radon exposure values were calculated for each miner from the date he began mining at Eldorado Nuclear mine to each sequential month of observation. These values were expressed as working level months (WLM), that is, the cumulative product of length of underground exposure in working months (170 h), and the concentration of radon daughters in working levels (one working level is equal to 1.3×10^5 MeV of potential alpha energy per liter of air) specific for the calendar year.

The two carcinogenic risk factors were quantitatively assessed as follows: the duration in years of cigarette smoking and the cigarette index were used to measure exposure to cigarette smoking; the duration in years of uranium mining and cumulative WLM were used to measure exposure to radon daughters.

Elliot Lake

In May of 1978, following a pilot project carried out by the Ontario Ministry of Labour, three of the authors (P. B., M. F., L. W.) initiated a sputum cytology program sponsored by the Elliot Lake Centre in three uranium mines in Ontario, two at Elliot Lake and one at Bancroft. The two Elliot Lake mines consist of the same ore body but are operated by different companies. Data collection and procedures were similar to those used in the Uranium City Project; sputum cytology evaluation was performed at the Banting Institute in Toronto. Individuals were invited to participate on a voluntary basis. For the first year of the study, participation was limited to "high risk" workers, namely workers in the crushing operation of the mill and to underground miners with any of the following: (1) mining experience of any duration prior to 1968, date from which improvement in mine ventilation occurred; (2) cumulative WLM of 100 or over; (3) mining experience of 5 years or more since 1968. By July 1978, the study became open to all workers. Since September 1979, a sputum cytology test became mandatory in the Province of Ontario for workers with at least 5 years of uranium mining experience. As a consequence, the sputum cytology study is now carried out at the Elliot Lake Centre in association with investigators from Ontario.

In this report, the data obtained during the first year of the survey in "high risk" *underground* uranium miners at Elliot Lake will be presented. Cumulative WLM values have not been completed for each miner and the duration of underground uranium mining is used as a measure of exposure.

Table 1. Uranium City Project: Marked atypia and cancer in "high risk" smoker underground uranium miners

Characteristics	Marked atypia	Cancer
Number	7	6
Mean age (years)	47	55
Mean years underground	16	13
Mean cumulative WLM	280	300
Mean years of cigarette smoking	25	36
Mean induction latent period (years)	18	21

Results

Uranium City Project

In-depth analysis of the results from the first 3 years of study has been recently reported [3]. Conclusions reached for underground uranium miners were as follows: (1) The overall observed frequency of abnormal cytology was 22% for smokers and 8% for nonsmokers ($p = 0.6$); (2) the estimated frequency of abnormal cytology among smokers was significantly dependent on the duration of cigarette smoking and of uranium mining; (3) the presence of both risk factors, smoking and exposure to radon daughters, resulted in a steady increase in the observed frequency of abnormal cytology linearly related to cumulative WLM exposure and to the number of years of uranium mining.

As of September 1980, seven individuals with marked atypia and six with lung cancer were observed among "high risk" smoker underground uranium miners (Table 1). Of the cancer patients, two were diagnosed prior to joining the survey; one had an oat cell tumor, the other a squamous cell carcinoma. Four patients were diagnosed during the survey. One, the only prevalence case, had an inoperable squamous cell carcinoma simultaneously detected by sputum cytology and chest X-ray and died 2 years after the diagnosis. Two patients developed oat cell carcinomas and died within 1 year of the diagnosis. In both, marked atypia was detected in sputum cytology specimens 13 and 24 months respectively previous to the first evidence of malignancy. The remaining patient had marked atypia for 6 months, followed by the development of an occult squamous cell carcinoma. This patient is alive and free of disease 5 years after the localization and surgical resection of a stage I tumor with negative lymph nodes. There were seven individuals in whom marked atypia was detected by sputum cytology.

Elliot Lake

The characteristics of the population studied and the distribution of cytology findings are shown in Tables 2 and 3 respectively. Mean age and years of underground mining experience were similar for both smokers and nonsmokers. However, the proportion of abnormal cytology findings, 48% and 5% for smokers and nonsmokers respectively, differed significantly ($p < 0.01$). Two patients with squamous cell lung carcinoma and six individuals with marked atypia were detected by sputum cytology (Table 4). At this time, follow-up is insufficient to assess the evolution of these cases.

Table 2. Elliot Lake: Characteristics of "high risk" underground uranium miners

Characteristics	Smoker	Nonsmoker
Number	132	21
Mean age (years)	45	44
Mean years underground	13	14
Mean years of cigarette smoking	23	0
Mean cigarette index	20	0

Table 3. Elliot Lake: Results of sputum cytology by smoking status

Cytology	Smoker		Nonsmoker	
	No.	%	No.	%
Normal and mild atypia	69	52	20	95
Moderate atypia	55	42	1	5
Marked atypia	6	4.5	0	0
Cancer	2	1.5	0	0
Total	132	100	21	100
Normal/abnormal[a]	63/132	48	1/21	5

[a] Smoker vs nonsmoker: $p < 0.1$

Table 4. Elliot Lake: Marked atypia and cancer in "high risk" smoker underground uranium miners

Characteristics	Marked atypia	Cancer
Number	6	2
Mean age (years)	45	57
Mean years underground	15	19
Mean years of cigarette smoking	26	37
Mean cigarette index	20	15
Mean induction latent period (years)	19	23

Discussion

The results of the Uranium City Project indicating a preponderance of abnormal sputum cytology findings among cigarette smoker underground uranium miners compared to nonsmokers [3] are confirmed by the preliminary data obtained in the high risk group of miners studied at Elliot Lake. Further, in both surveys, severe atypical squamous cell metaplasia (marked atypia) was only observed among smokers. Sputum cytology studies of uranium miners [11], and of non-uranium miners [7, 8] have suggested that markedly atypical squamous cells may be precursors to malignancy. This indication is supported by the findings of Kato et al. (this

Symposium); these authors observed, in a lung cancer experimental model induced in dogs by 20-methylcholanthrene injection into the bronchial submucosa, the development of severe atypical squamous cell metaplasia prior to the occurrence of in situ carcinoma.

In the Uranium City Project, 10 individuals with marked atypia were observed. They were exhaustively followed with sputum cytology *and* selective fiberoptic bronchoscopy at 3-month intervals for 3 years, and with monthly sputum cytology thereafter. In three cases a bronchogenic cancer was detected, after an observation periods of 6, 13, and 24 months respectively. This 30% incidence of lung cancer supports the view that marked atypia may represent a preneoplastic condition. The remaining seven individuals, however, have all "reverted" to lesser degrees of atypia, despite continued cigarette smoking and uranium mining, during a mean follow-up period of 60 months (range 24–72 months).

The characteristics of the high risk underground uranium miners from the Uranium City and Elliot Lake surveys (Tables 1 and 4) are remarkably similar and reveal and induction latent periods to marked atypia of 18 years (range 10–22 years) and of 19 years (range 11–22 years) respectively.

Based on the above results and experience, the following suggestions are tentatively offered. Sputum cytology surveys of uranium miners may be confined to high risk workers with screening initiated, for a given miner, 10 years after his first occupational exposure to radiation. Individuals with marked atypias may be followed with twice yearly sputum cytology and selective segmental fiberoptic bronchoscopy for 2 years and with twice yearly cytology for an additional 2 years or longer if marked atypia persists.

The value of sputum cytology in the early detection of lung cancer is currently being assessed in various high risk groups. Preliminary results indicate a prolonged survival in the subgroup of patients with squamous cell carcinoma detected by sputum cytology alone. Although no such effect has been observed in small cell carcinoma, advances in the treatment of this disease [13] might improve results in occult cases.

In view of recent developments in cancer chemoprophylaxis with retinoids [4, 12], the role of sputum cytology in the prevention of lung cancer should become a preponderant aspect of screening programs. Well designed large surveys of high risk groups provide at this time the only means to determine quantitatively the proportion of moderate and marked atypias with an evolutionary potential to malignancy. However, the full impact of sputum cytology in the prevention of lung cancer will depend on a better characterization of marked atypia in order to discriminate beforehand those which are committed to develop into cancer. It has been shown that a majority of atypical squamous metaplastic cells have a heteroploid DNA distribution pattern similar to in situ cancer cells [9; Nasiell et al.; Kato et al., this Symposium]. Whether this characteristic is confined to marked atypia with a neoplastic potential needs to be assessed prospectively. Of added interest are the observations of Balchum, Hayata, King, and their respective colleagues (this Symposium) indicating that foci of atypical metaplasia may be localized by fluorescence bronchoscopy using hematoporphyrin derivative. These areas, once localized, could be treated endobronchially with phototherapy.

Fluorescence bronchoscopy, phototherapy, chemoprophylaxis, and adjuvant therapy of small cell carcinoma represent recent technical and therapeutic advances which add new dimensions to the role of sputum cytology in the prevention and early detection of lung cancer.

References

1. Archer VE, Wagoner JK (1973) Lung cancer among uranium miners in the United States. Health Phys 25: 351–371
2. Archer VE, Gillam JD, Wagoner JK (1976) Respiratory disease mortality among uranium miners. Ann NY Acad Sci 271: 280–293
3. Band PR, Feldstein M, Saccomanno G, Watson L, King G (1980) Potentiation of cigarette smoking and radiation: evidence from a sputum cytology survey among uranium miners and controls. Cancer 45: 1273–1277
4. Bollag W (1979) Retinoids and cancer. Cancer Chemother Pharmacol 3: 207–215
5. Hueper WC (1966) Occupational and environmental cancers of the respiratory system. Recent Results Cancer Res 3: 125–147
6. Lundin FE, Wagoner JK, Archer VE (1971) Radon daughter exposure and respiratory cancer: quantitative and temporal aspects. NIOSH and NIESH Joint Monograph No 1. National Technical Information Service, Springfield
7. Nasiell M (1966) Metaplasia and atypical metaplasia in the bronchial epithelium: a histopathologic and cytopathologic study. Acta Cytol (Baltimore) 10: 421–427
8. Nasiell M (1976) Cytology of benign changes and carcinoma in situ of the lung. In: Wied GL, Koss LG, Reagan JW (eds) Tutorials of cytology. Tutorial proceedings of the International Academy of Cytology: Compendium on Diagnostic Cytology, 6th edn, vol IV. Chicago, Illinois, pp 315–329
9. Nasiell M, Kato H, Auer G, Zetterberg A, Roger V, Karlen L (1978) Cytomorphological grading and feulgen DNA-analysis of metaplastic and neoplastic bronchial cells. Cancer 41: 1511–1521
10. Saccomanno G, Saunders RP, Archer VE, Auerbach O, Kuschner M, Beckler PA (1965) Cancer of the lung: the cytology of sputum prior to the development of carcinoma. Acta Cytol (Balitmore) 9: 413–423
11. Saccomanno G, Archer VE, Auerbach O, Saunders RP, Brennan LM (1974) Development of carcinoma of the lung as reflected in exfoliated cells. Cancer 33: 256–270
12. Sporn MB, Dunlop NM, Newton DN, Smith JM (1976) Prevention of chemical carcinogenesis by Vitamin A and its synthetic analogs (retinoids). Fed Proc 35: 1332–1338
13. Vincent RG, Wilson HE, Lane WW et al. (1981) Progress in the chemotherapy of small cell carcinoma of the lung. Cancer 47: 229–235
14. Wagoner JK, Archer VE, Lundir FE, Holaday DA, Lloyd JW (1965) Radiation as the cause of lung cancer among uranium miners. N Engl J Med 273: 181–188
15. Wynder EL (1972) Etiology of lung cancer. Reflections on two decades of research. Cancer 30: 1332–1339

*Detection of Early and Roentgenologically
Occult Bronchogenic Carcinoma:
Preliminary Report of the Sabbatsberg Hospital
Sputum Cytologic Screening Study*

M. Nasiell, J. Kinnman, S. Haglund, V. Roger, and K. Nasiell

Sabbatsberg Hospital, Departments of Pathology and Cytology, Box 6401,
S-133 82 Stockholm, Sweden

Introduction

A sputum cytologic screening project aiming at early diagnosis and study of the
pathogenesis of bronchogenic carcinoma has been going on at Sabbatsberg Hospital,
Stockholm, since 1964. In 1974 the project was reorganized to study a target
population of male cigarette smokers without known lung disease at high cancer risk
from outpatient clinics and various companies and organizations [1].

Materials and Methods

Three early morning cough specimens (3 × 4 slides) are carefully examined by
specially trained cytotechnologists using detailed cytomorphologic criteria for the
various epithelial abnormalities. Cytologic evidence of early epithelial injury
(abnormal columnar cell finding – ACCF) [2], various degrees of atypical squamous
metaplasia (mild, moderate, and severe) [4], evidence of early bronchial carcinoma
(carcinoma in situ or early invasive carcinoma), and outspoken cancer [3] are recorded
on the patients' charts. In addition, archival material has been used for determining
the biological significance of the epithelial atypias by retrospective quantitative
measurements of the DNA content of "premalignant" cell changes [4]. The routine
clinical procedures during this prevalence cytology screening study are shown in Fig. 1.
Localization of clinically occult lesions is performed with fiberoptic bronchoscopy by
the participating otolaryngologists who also make a routine ENT examination to
exclude malignancies in the upper respiratory and alimentary passages. The
otolaryngologists (J.K. and S.H.), in addition, perform mediastinoscopy in those
patients who are candidates for surgical resection. During this phase of the screening
study only sputum cytology has been used as the primary detection method. Smokers
with positive cytology were referred for further investigation including X-ray and
fiberoptic bronchoscopy [1].
The screening material consists of 3,042 men, over 45 years of age, who have smoked
20 cigarettes per day for 15 years or more. We also examined patients from a routine
clinical material with chest X-rays that showed no changes indicating lung
cancer.

Recent Results in Cancer Research, Vol. 82
© Springer-Verlag Berlin · Heidelberg 1982

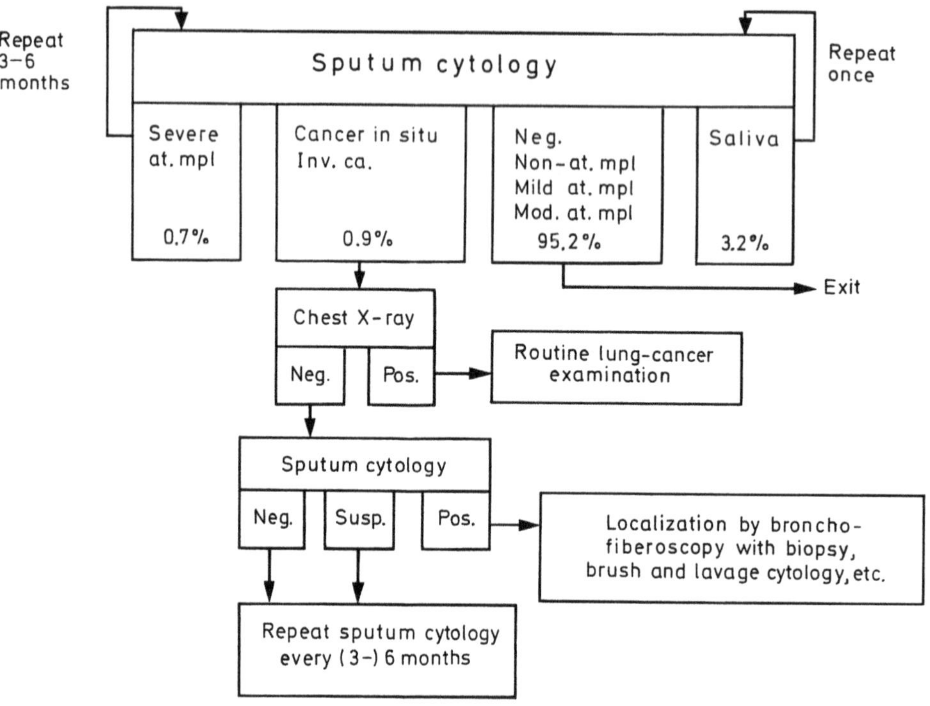

Fig. 1. Sabbatsberg Hospital sputum cytology screening study for early bronchogenic carcinoma in high risk smokers. Procedures and results (May 1980)

Results and Conclusions

Among the high risk smokers, 28 (0.9%) had positive or highly suspicious cytology — 23 were clinically occult carcinomas (Fig. 1, Table 1). In the clinical routine material 60 patients with evidence of clinically occult cancer were found.

Fiberoptic bronchoscopy has been used since 1974—1975 in Stockholm and so far (May 1980) 28 out of altogether 83 (23 + 60) clinically occult bronchogenic carcinomas have been localized in the total material (screening *and* clinical material). Twenty-two of these underwent surgical treatment (Table 2).

Average age at surgery was 61 years (range 48—71) and the average follow-up time more than 3 years (May 1980). Eighteen of the 22 patients were operated on in the period 1975—1980. This increasing activity indicates a clinical consciousness of the present possibilities of early detection (sputum cytology) and localization (fiberoptic bronchoscopy) of occult early and operable bronchogenic cancer. During this later period of the project the time lapse from the first positive cytological finding to resection was on an average 3 months (range 1—7 months).

Among the 61 nonresected patients in the total material, 20 mainly pertaining to the early part of the series from 1964 to 1974, died *from lung cancer* even though the tumor had been diagnosed cytologically before it produced positive radiological changes (Table 3). Fifteen patients died of intercurrent disease. In 24 cases definite diagnosis is still lacking (May 1980).

Table 1. Twenty-eight cytologically positive cases in the screening material (August 1975–May 1980)

Cytology indicating early squamous cell cancer	23
Resected	11 (40%)
Localized but inoperable	1
Later dead from lung cancer intercurrent disease	5
Follow-up	6
Other malignant cytologic findings	5
Advanced squamous cell lung cancer/adenocarcinoma	3
Larynx carcinoma	2
Total	28

Table 2. Resected cases – Total material

No sign of recurrence	15[a] (68%)
Dead from lung cancer	5
Dead from intercurrent disease	2
Total	22

[a] Atypia or carcinoma in situ in resection border

Table 3. Sputum cytologic diagnosis of early lung cancer – Nonresected

	Total material	Histol. verif. carcinoma in situ[a]	Histol. verif. invasive carcinoma	Cytol. diagn. only
Dead from invasive cancer	20	4	16	0
Dead from intercurrent disease	15	3	0	12
Localized but inoperable	2	0	2	0
Follow-up cases	24	0	0	24
Total	61	7	18	36

[a] ± early stromal invasion

The results indicate that with increasing experience and more active clinical diagnostic procedures, early bronchogenic carcinoma can be detected and localized by sputum cytology and fiberoptic bronchoscopy, which gives hope for a more successful treatment of the disease.

Prevalence screening has a tendency to detect cases with a relatively long preclinical duration and a correspondingly slow growth. The end result will be determined by the total lung cancer deaths. Two main questions remain and will be the subject for further studies:

1) Does early diagnosis influence the natural course of squamous cell bronchogenic carcinoma?
2) How many additional bronchogenic carcinomas (incidence cases) can be expected to develop in the screening material?

References

1. Haglund S, Kinnman J, Malmström L, Nasiell K, Nasiell M, Roger V (1979) The Sabbatsberg Hospital sputum cytologic study of roentgenologically occult bronchial cancer. Lakartidningen 76: 735–738
2. Nasiell M (1967) Abnormal columnar cell findings in bronchial epithelium. A cytologic and histologic study of lung cancer and non-cancer cases. Acta Cytol (Baltimore) 11: 397–402
3. Nasiell M, Sinner W, Tornvall G (1977) Clinically occult lung cancer with positive sputum cytology and primarily negative roentgenologic findings. Scand J Respir Dis 58: 134–144
4. Nasiell M, Kato H, Auer G, Zetterberg A, Roger V, Karlen L (1978) Cytomorphological grading and Feulgen DNA-analysis of metaplastic and neoplastic bronchial cells. Cancer 41: 1511–1521

Results of Lung Cancer Screening Programs in Japan*

Y. Hayata, H. Funatsu, H. Kato, Y. Saito, K. Sawamura, and K. Furose

Tokyo Medical College, Department of Surgery, 6-7-1, Nishishinjuku, Shinjuku-ku,
J-Tokyo 160 Japan

Introduction

In 1953 we began in Japan a lung cancer detection program by chest X-ray surveys
amongst several groups including employees of the Tokyo Metropolitan Government
(TMG). The results obtained from this 27-year survey indicate that chest X-rays are
effective in the detection of early stage lung cancer located peripherally but not
centrally in the lung. At the Department of Surgery, Tokyo Medical College, 54 cases
of early stage lung cancer were treated; 45 cases were peripheral and only nine cases
were central. Of the nine centrally located tumors only two (22%) were detected by
chest X-ray survey, as opposed to 71% of the peripheral-type cases similarly detected.
Sputum cytology surveys have thus gained increasing attention in Japan for the
detection of early stage central lung cancer, particularly in cases where the chest X-ray
is negative. A sputum cytology study is thus being conducted amongst high risk
employees of the TMG as well as amongst local residents of the Itabashi area in Tokyo
aged 40 years and over, but the results are as yet inconclusive. However, in addition to
detecting early stage lung cancer, the objective of sputum cytology surveys should
include the detection of atypical squamous cell metaplasia, since this condition has
been shown experimentally [Kato et al., this Symposium] and clinically [1, 17, 18, 21]
to be involved in the development of squamous cell carcinoma. Squamous cell
metaplasia is therefore checked for in our survey cases, and chronological changes of
nuclear atypia are monitored. Our chest X-ray survey of employees of the TMG is a
representative study that has been carried out over a long period of time. There are
several other groups conducting sputum cytology and/or chest X-ray surveys in Japan,
particularly the National Kinki Central Hospital Group, where two of us (K.S. and
K.F.) have initiated a chest X-ray and sputum cytology project which has yielded a
high rate of lung cancer detection.

Materials and Methods

Chest X-ray Survey of Employees of TMG

A total of 1,871,374 examinations were made between 1953 and 1979 using
posteroanterior chest roentgenograms. Prior to 1969, 35- or 60-mm films were used,

---

* Supported in part by a Grant-in-Aid for Cancer Research from the Ministry of Health and
Welfare and the Tokyo Medical College Cancer Centre

whereas 70- or 100-mm films have been used since then. Examinations were conducted annually with the exception of certain special groups which were examined semiannually. Cases in which abnormal findings were recognized were generally referred to the Department of Surgery, Tokyo Medical College, for investigation and treatment.

Sputum Cytology Survey of Employees of TMG

Since 1975, a total of 4,212 high risk individuals were asked to send one sputum specimen annually. An individual is considered to be in a high risk group if he or she is at least 40 years old and a heavy smoker (20 cigarettes/day), or has a persistent cough or bloody sputum. Sputum specimens from three to five consecutive deep cough expectorations obtained upon arising are pooled in a transparent vinyl bag containing 50% methyl alcohol and 1% thymol. The bag is then placed in a special container and sent to our laboratory by mail. The containers were made according to the specifications of the Department of Surgery, Tokyo Medical College, and are $9.5 \times 6.0 \times 1.6$ cm in size.

Sputum Cytology Survey of Local Residents in the Itabashi Area in Tokyo

This survey was carried out on a total of 1,025 participants of both sexes aged 40 years and over; sputum specimens were obtained as described above.
In both of these groups (TMG and Itabashi residents), squamous cell metaplasia as well as cancer cells were looked for. The cytologic material was graded according to Nasiell's [17] and Saccomanno's [21] criteria for atypical squamous cell metaplastia.

Lung Cancer Screening by the National Kinki Central Hospital Group

Between 1975 and 1979, 178,295 individuals underwent screening with chest X-ray or sputum cytology once or twice a year. All were aged 40 years or over, and belonged to a wide spectrum of environmental or occupational populations. Consequently, the purpose and the number of screening procedures differed according to each subgroup (Table 1). Sputum samples were assessed using the Saccomanno method [21].

Table 1. National Kinki Central Hospital Group survey participants

Examinees	Purpose of survey	Number of yearly examinations
Local residents	Pulmonary tuberculosis	1–2
Labor union members	Pulmonary tuberculosis	1–2
Environmental pollution	Chronic bronchitis	1
Occupational pollution	Chronic bronchitis	1–2
Complete physicals on short hospitalization	Any abnormality	1
Physical checkups for adult diseases	Various diseases	1
Lung cancer	Lung cancer	1
Newly admitted elderly man with tuberculosis	Lung cancer	–

Results

Chest X-ray Survey of Employees of TMG

Over the 27-year course of this survey, 193 lung cancer cases were detected among a total of 1,871,374 examinations, an overall ratio of 10.3 per 100,000. However, the lung cancer detection rate for men aged 40 years or over was almost three times that for women in the same category (Table 2), and 82.3% of all lung cancer cases were detected among individuals of 50 years or over (Table 3). Of the 193 cases, the tumor

Table 2. Discovery rate of lung cancer by chest X-ray mass survey according to sex and age of employees of Tokyo Metropolitan Government (1953–1979)

Sex	Age	Examinations	Lung cancer cases	
			Number	Rate per 100,000
Male	Total	1,370,636	172	12.5
	40 and over	603,597	169	28.0
Female	Total	500,738	21	4.2
	40 and over	177,009	19	10.7
Total		1,871,374	193	10.3
	40 and over	780,606	188	24.1

Table 3. Age distribution of lung cancer detected by chest X-ray survey (Tokyo Metropolitan Government)

Age	No. of examinations	Lung cancer cases	
		Number	Rate per 100,000
<39	1,090,768	5	0.5
40–49	427,784	27	6.3
50–59	254,018	62	24.4
60 and over	98,804	99	100.2
Total	1,871,374	193	10.3

Table 4. Breakdown of lung cancer cases detected by chest X-ray survey according to location and stage of the tumor (Tokyo Metropolitan Government)

Tumor location	No.	Stage I		Stage II		Stage III		Stage IV	
		No.	%	No.	%	No.	%	No.	%
Central	81	16	(19.8)[a]	13	(16.0)	31	(38.3)	21	(26.9)
Peripheral	112	65	(58.0)[a]	14	(12.5)	22	(19.6)	11	(9.8)

[a] $p < 0.001$

Table 5. Early stage lung cancer detection according to intervals between surveys (Tokyo Metropolitan Government)

Group[a]	Total number of lung cancer cases	Early stage cancer	
		No.	%
1	32	9	28.1
2	94	9	9.6
3	67	6	9.0

Group 1: 2, $p < 0.03$; Group 1: 3, $p < 0.03$; Group 2: $p < 0.9$

[a] Group 1: Semiannual examination on workers in harmful environments, night workers, and workers with a history of pulmonary tuberculosis
Group 2: Annual examination on office workers
Group 3: Not examined the previous year or overlooked or misdiagnosed in the previous year's examination

Table 6. Comparison of resectability and 5-year survival between the surveyed (TMG) and the nonsurveyed cases treated at the department of surgery, Tokyo Medical College

Group	Total number of lung cancer cases	Resectability		5-year survival[a]	
		No.	%		
Survey	193	108	(56.0)	34/78[a]	(43.6)
Nonsurvey	1,156	353	(30.5)	48/236[a]	(20.3)
	$p < 0.001$	$p < 0.001$		$p < 0.001$	

[a] Number surviving 5 years over the total number of cases resected 5 years ago or earlier

location was central in 81 and peripheral in 112, but for stage I tumors only 19.8% were central whereas 58% were in the periphery of the lungs (Table 4). Comparing the clinical stage of detected cases with the interval between examinations, the percentage of early stage lung cancer was 28.1% in the semiannual examination group (group 1), 9.6% in the annual group (group 2), and 9.0% in group 3 (not examined, or overlooked, or misdiagnosed the previous year), as is shown in Table 5.

Resectability and 5-year survival were compared between cases from the TMG surveyed group and nonsurveyed cases treated at our institution: resectability was 56% and 30.5%, and the 5-year survival was 43.6% and 20.3%, respectively, in the former and latter groups (Table 6), a statistically significant difference, for both resectability and survival. When resectability and survival were compared in terms of interval between surveys (Table 7), a statistically significant difference was shown for resectability in group 1 (90.6%), but no difference in survival was apparent between the three groups. However, the postoperative cancer death rate in curatively resected cases was significantly lower ($p < 0.02$) in the surveyed group (34.1%) than the nonsurveyed group (56.3%).

Table 7. Resectability and 5-year survival according to interval of survey (Tokyo Metropolitan Government)

Group[a]	Number of lung cancer cases	Resectability		5-year survival[b]	
		No.	%		
1	32	29	90.6	10/18	(55.5)
2	94	50	53.2	18/39	(46.2)
3	67	29	43.3	6/21	(28.6)

Resectability: Group 1: 2, $p < 0.001$; Group 1: 3, $p < 0.001$; Group 2: 3, $p < 0.3$
5-Year survival: Group 1: 2, $p < 0.6$; Group 1: 3, $p < 0.08$; Group 2: 3, $p < 0.2$
[a] See Table 5
[b] See Table 6

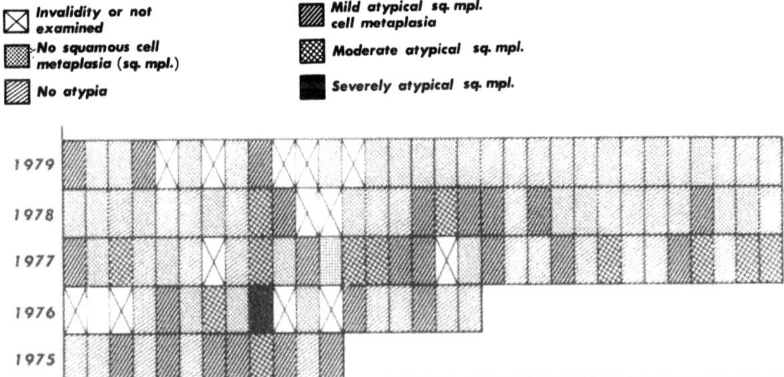

Fig. 1. Chronological changes of nuclear atypia in squamous cell metaplasia cases detected by sputum cytology survey on high risk group of Tokyo Metropolitan Government employees

Sputum Cytology Survey of Employees of TMG

Although containers to collect specimens were distributed to 4,212 individuals in the high risk group, only 2,100 (49.8%) returned them, and of these only 1,167 (56.6%) gave valid samples. No lung cancer was detected, but squamous cell metaplasia was found in 40.4% of the cases (Table 8). We followed the chronological changes of nuclear atypia in the TMG cases in which squamous metaplasia was detected (Fig. 1). The degree of nuclear atypia increased in four cases and decreased in 23. No case developed to carcinoma in situ or early stage carcinoma.

Sputum Cytology Survey in the Itabashi Area

Containers for specimen collection were issued to 1,025 persons, but the number of specimens returned was 682 (66.3%). Of these, 564 (82.9%) were valid samples. One case was discovered with negative chest X-ray, but positive sputum cytology. Squamous cell metaplasia was found in 325 cases, but no relation was observed between the cigarette index and the degree of atypia (Table 9).

Table 8. Results of sputum cytology survey in the high risk group in relation to smoking index and nuclear atypia of squamous cell metaplasia (Tokyo Metropolitan Government)

Cigarette index	Number of samples returned	Valid samples		Number of squamous cell metaplasia					Squamous cell metaplasia	
		No.	%	None	Regular	Mild	Moderate	Severe	No./Total	%
0	412	217	42.7	142	55	17	4	0	76/217	(35.0)
1–400	699	364	52.1	218	113	25	8	0	146/364	(40.1)
401–800	696	406	58.3	241	119	41	5	1	166/406	(40.9)
801 or more	294	180	61.2	96	61	19	3	1	84/180	(46.7)
Total	2,100	1,167	55.6	697	348	102	20	2	472/1,167	(40.4)

Total number of individuals given specimen containers: 4,212

Table 9. Results of sputum cytology survey in the local residents of Itabashi area in relation to smoking index and nuclear atypia of squamous cell metaplasia (1978)

Cigarette index	Number of samples returned	Valid samples		Number of squamous cell metaplasia					Lung cancer	Squamous cell metaplasia	
		No.	%	None	Regular	Mild	Mod-erate	Severe		No./total	%
0	221	169	76.4	83	65	12	7	2	0	86/169	(50.8)
1–400	185	150	81.1	61	62	26	1	0	0	89/150	(59.3)
401–800	187	169	90.4	64	77	26	2	0	0	105/169	(62.1)
801 or more	87	76	87.4	30	30	12	3	0	1	45/76	(59.2)
Total	680	564	82.9	238	234	76	13	2	1	325/564	(57.6)

Total number of individuals given specimen containers: 1,025

Table 10. Discovery rate of lung cancer by mass survey according to group of examinees (National Kinki Central Hospital Group, 1975–1979)

Group of examinees	Number of examinees	Incidence of high risk	Percent sputum cytology performed	Number of lung cancer detected	Number of early lung cancer	Lung cancer rate per 100,000
Local residents	91,486	3.4%	0.1	8	0	8.7
Labor union members	30,388	36.4%	7.4	3	1	9.9
Environmental pollution	3,715	12.4%	51.2	5	1	134.6
Occupational pollution	825	38.1%	87.9	2	1	242.1
Complete physicals on short hospitalization	6,309	48.7%	52.9	13	3	206.1
Physical checkup for adult disease	24,155	68.3%	1.5	15	3	62.1
Lung cancer	21,038	29.5%	12.4	17	5	80.8
Newly admitted elderly man with tuberculosis	342	97.1%	100.0	11	2	3,216.4
Total	178,259	23.0%	6.5	74	16	41.5

Table 11. Analysis of lung cancer detected by chest X-ray and sputum cytology according to tumor location and histology (National Kinki Central Hospital Group)

	Number of lung cancers detected	
	Chest X-ray	Sputum cytology
Central tumors	7	22
Squamous cell carcinoma	14	27
Adenocarcinoma	21	4
Large cell carcinoma	2	0
Small cell carcinoma	4	1
Other histology	1	0
Early stage carcinoma	5	11
Total	42	32

Table 12. Comparison of resectability between surveyed and nonsurveyed group (National Kinki Central Hospital Group)

Resectability	Survey group		Nonsurvey group	
	No.	%	No.	%
Curative	22	29.7[a]	85	13.0
Noncurative	12	16.2	103	15.9
Inoperable	40	54.9	464	71.1
Total	74		652	

[a] $p < 0.001$

Table 13. Percent 3-year survival between surveyed and nonsurveyed group (National Kinki Central Hospital Group)

Resection	Survey	Nonsurvey
Curative	92.6	70.1
Noncurative	33.3	11.0

National Kinki Central Hospital Group Survey

Lung cancer was detected in 74 individuals out of a total of 178,295 examinees, an overall detection rate of 41.5 per 100,000, and sputum cytology was performed in 6.5% of all cases (Table 10). Amongst the 74 lung cancer cases, 42 were detected by chest X-ray and 32 by sputum cytology; 16 were early stage lung cancer. Half of the cases detected by chest X-ray were adenocarcinomas, whereas almost 85% of those diagnosed by sputum cytology were squamous cell carcinomas (Table 11). Thirty-four cases were resected, while the remaining 40 cases were not operated, because of age, advanced stage of the disease, other illnesses, or refusal of surgery. However, the surveyed group had a better resectability rate (Table 12) and a better 3-year survival rate (Table 13) than the nonsurveyed group; also there were fewer postoperative deaths in the curatively resected survey cases (4.5%), as compared to 24.7% in the nonsurveyed group resected for cancer ($p < 0.05$).

Discussion

Chest X-ray survey for the detection of lung cancer is a law in Japan and is carried out by local agencies and by employers. Therefore the chest X-ray detection of lung cancer may be obtained in Japan at no extra cost, and since Overholt's report [19], chest X-ray surveys have been performed to detect both tuberculosis and lung cancer. Summarizing the detection rates of lung cancer by chest X-ray surveys in Japan, the overall rate per 100,000 ranged from 3.0 to 20.5, and from 15.3 to 29.0 for individuals aged 40 years or over, with higher rates in special occupational populations. These results do not significantly differ from those of the chest X-ray surveys carried out in the United States and in Europe where the lung cancer detection rates ranged from 3.4 to 11.9 [2, 9, 10, 13, 14, 19]. However, in high risk groups or groups of subjects aged 40 years or over the lung cancer detection rates per 100,000 increased from 33.8 up to 74.4 [3, 16, 20].
Our results at the Department of Surgery, Tokyo Medical College, of the chest X-ray survey of employees of the TMG showed an overall lung cancer detection rate of 10.3 per 100,000 and of 24.1 for the age group 40 years and over; these represent standard rates for workers in Japan and do not compare with the overall lung cancer detection rate of 41.5 per 100,000 observed by the National Kinki Central Hospital Group. The discrepancy between the results obtained at these two institutions is attributed to differences in the types of population surveyed. In particular, groups at high risk of developing lung cancer because of exposure to environmental or occupational pollution factors were included in the National Kinki Central Hospital Study. It would thus appear that in order to improve the yield of lung cancer detection by chest X-ray, this procedure should be performed amongst city residents or workers at least 40−45 years old. However, for more efficient lung cancer discovery rates, stricter candidate selection is necessary. For instance, Kubik [11] discovered 61 cases of lung cancer among 12,322 examinees aged 40−64 years who were heavy smokers or complained of cough or had a history of pulmonary diseases. Also, the lung cancer rate reached 242.1 per 100,000 in the high risk group studied at the National Kinki Central Hospital. It will be necessary to study a given high risk group for prolonged periods of time to detect many lung cancers.
The time interval between chest X-ray surveys should be looked at in terms of the results of resectability as well as survival and detection rates of early stage lung cancer. With regard to the former, Brett [5] has indicated a higher resectability rate in surveyed cases than in a control group; the results of our studies confirm this observation. Concerning survival, Boucot and Weiss [4] failed to find a significant difference in 5-year survival between chest X-ray surveyed and nonsurveyed patients. However, among the employees of the TMG, the overall 5-year survival was 20.6%, as opposed to 5.3% for the nonsurveyed patients treated at the Department of Surgery, Tokyo Medical College. The 3-year survival rate of 26 resected cases amongst 200

patients surveyed was reported to be 12% by Lilienfield et al. [12]. However, in 78 TMG resected cases detected 5 years ago, or earlier, the 5-year survival was 43.6%, as compared to 20.3% for 236 nonsurveyed patients resected at the Department of Surgery, Tokyo Medical College. In the TMG chest X-ray survey, the rate of detection of early stage lung cancer was 28.1% when examination was carried out semiannually, but only 9.6% in individuals examined on a yearly basis; however, the 5-year survival of these resected patients did not differ significantly, being 55.5% and 46.2% respectively. The significant differences in resectability and survival of resected cases between our patients and those of Lilienfield et al. [12] are probably related to differences in histologic type, tumor location, and interval from diagnosis to treatment; most TMG patients were treated within 3 months of detection. When expense and cost-effectiveness are considered, chest X-ray surveys should be performed in specific high risk groups as indicated by the American Cancer Society (ACS). However, chest X-ray surveys should be performed more widely for high risk groups aged 40 years and over in order to obtain maximum detection of lung cancer, and semiannual examinations appear to be the best method available to detect early peripheral lung cancer. These considerations also apply to sputum cytology surveys.

Sputum cytology surveys are essential to detect centrally located lung cancer when the lesion is occult. Among 193 cases of lung cancer detected in the TMG survey, there was only one central-type early stage lung cancer. We have therefore initiated a sputum cytology survey in the high risk groups of the TMG employees and among the Itabashi residents in Tokyo, but so far only one early lung cancer has been detected. The National Kinki Central Hospital Group has treated 30 cases of early central-type lung cancer, of which 12 were patients with normal chest X-ray diagnosed by sputum cytology. Fontana [6, 7], Weiss [22], Melamed [15], Grzybowski [8], and their respective colleagues have reported their results with sputum cytology survey, and have recognized its value to detect occult lung cancer. Despite the controversy raised by the ACS concerning sputum cytology surveys, we feel that these surveys should be continued for high risk groups. Concerning the ACS comments on the Mayo Lung Project, we feel that it is much too early to evaluate this vast and excellently designed project, as the 5-year survival figures currently available represent cases diagnosed during the first 3−4 years of the project (after the prevalence cases were excluded) and might well encompass the most rapidly proliferating tumors rather than the more slowly proliferating tumors one may encounter over a longer study period.

The necessity of following up individuals with atypical squamous cell metaplasia to detect lung cancer has been emphasized [1, 18, 21]. In our canine lung cancer model [Kato et al., this Symposium], we observed in all cases increasing degrees of atypical squamous cell metaplasia prior to the development of squamous cell carcinoma. The role of chronologic sputum cytology follow-up of individuals with squamous cell metaplasia needs to be further elucidated with regard to the prevention and early detection of lung cancer. One of the basic problems in sputum cytology surveys is that of obtaining a high percentage of valid specimens and a good patient compliance. In order to improve our low rates of sputum cytology return and specimen validity, we published a pamphlet based on the one produced by Band and his colleagues. All individuals surveyed are now given a copy of this pamphlet together with the sputum container.

Recently, the incidence of adenocarcinoma of the lung has shown a tendency to increase throughout the world. Thus, the importance of chest X-ray surveys should be stressed for the detection of peripheral early lung cancer. To conclude, we feel that both chest X-ray and sputum cytology surveys have an important role to play in mass screening of high risk groups for the detection of lung cancer and hence in improving the survival rates among patients.

References

1. Band P, Feldstein M, Saccomanno G, Watson L, King G (1980) Potentiation of cigarette smoking and radiation. Evidence from a sputum cytology survey among uranium miners and controls. Cancer 45: 1273–1277
2. Bondi G, Leites V (1952) Malignant neoplastic disease discovered in chest X-ray survey. N Engl J Med 247: 506–512
3. Boucot KR, Sokoloff MJ (1954) Preclinical bronchogenic carcinoma. Am Rev. Tuberc 69: 164–172
4. Boucot KR, Weiss W (1973) Is curable lung cancer detected by semi-annual screening? JAMA 224: 1361–1365
5. Brett GZ (1968) The value of lung cancer detection by six-monthly chest radiographs. Thorax 23: 414–420
6. Fontana RS (1977) Early diagnosis of lung cancer. Am Rev Respir Dis 116: 399–402
7. Fontana RS, Sanderson DR, Woolner LB et al. (1975) The Mayo lung project for detection and localization of bronchogenic carcinoma: a status report. Chest 67: 511–522
8. Grzybowski S, Coy P (1970) Early diagnosis of carcinoma of the lung. Simultaneous screening with chest X-ray and sputum cytology. Cancer 25: 113–120
9. Guiss LW (1955) Mass roentgenographic screening as a lung-cancer-control measure. Cancer 8: 210–236
10. Honold R (1954) Früherfassung von Lungenkarzinomen durch das Schirmbild. Schweiz Med Wochenschr 84: 431–439
11. Kubik A, Křivinka R, Stašek V et al. (1970) Screening for lung cancer high-risk groups. Scand J Respir Dis 51: 290–300
12. Lilienfeld A, Archer PG, Burnett CH et al (1966) An evaluation of radiologic and cytologic screening for the early detection of lung cancer: a cooperative pilot study of the American Cancer Society and the Veterans Administration. Cancer Res 26: 2082–2121
13. McClure CD (1957) Followup study of 844 neoplasm suspects identified in a mass chest X-ray survey. Public Health Rep 72: 307–316
14. McNalti JM (1954) Clinical follow-up study of 398 patients suspected of having lung cancer discovered in the Boston chest X-ray survey. N Engl J Med 250: 14–17
15. Melamed M, Flehinger B, Miller D et al. (1977) Preliminary report of the lung cancer detection program in New York. Cancer 39: 369–382
16. Nash FA, Morgan JM, Tomkins JG (1968) South London cancer study. Br Med J 22: 715–721
17. Nasiell M (1967) Abnormal columnar cell findings in bronchial epithelium. A cytological and histologic study of lung cancer and non-lung cancer cases. Acta Cytol (Baltimore) 11: 397–402
18. Nasiell M, Sinner W, Tornvall G, Roger V, Vorel B, Enstad I (1977) Clinically occult lung cancer with positive sputum cytology and primarily negative radiological findings. Scand J Respir Dis 58: 134–144
19. Overholt RH (1950) Cancer detected in surveys. Am Rev Tuberc 62: 491–500
20. Posner E, McDowell LA, Cross KW (1963) Place of mass radiography in relation to lung cancer in men. Br Med J 9: 1156–1160
21. Saccomanno G, Archer VC, Auerbach O, Saunders RP, Brennan LM (1974) Development of carcinoma of the lung as reflected in exfoliated cells. Cancer 33: 256–270
22. Weiss W, Seidman H, Boucot KR (1978) The Philadelphia pulmonary neoplasm research project symptoms in occult lung cancer. Chest 73: 57–61

Results of the Memorial Sloan-Kettering Lung Project

N. Martini

Memorial Sloan-Kettering Cancer Center, Cornell University Medical College,
New York, NY, USA

The New York lung cancer detection program is part of the cooperative study initiated at Johns Hopkins Hospital and at the Mayo Clinic, and supported by the National Cancer Institute [2, 8, 9, 11]. We began screening in 1974, and over a period of 3 $^1/_2$ years, 10,040 men were entered into the program. All were 45 years of age or older, and smoked one or more packs of cigarettes a day for over 20 years.

Each person had a posteroanterior and lateral chest X-ray at his initial visit and yearly chest X-rays thereafter. One half of the screenees also had sputum cytologic examinations at 4-month intervals. The majority of those suspected of lung cancer underwent further evaluation and treatment at Memorial Hospital.

There have been 169 lung cancers found to date among the 10,040 entered into the study [10]. Fifty-five were discovered at initial examination, a prevalence rate of 5.5 per thousand; 114 additional cancers were detected on follow-up, an incidence rate of 3 per thousand per year. All cancers were clinically staged before treatment according to the AJC staging system [12]. Except for those with clinically evident distant metastases and those considered a major risk for surgery, all patients were recommended thoracotomy. Enlarged hilar or ipsilateral mediastinal lymph nodes were not considered contraindications to surgical treatment. When the surgery was performed at Memorial Hospital an effort was made to accurately assess the mediastinum for metastases at the time of the thoracotomy. When resection was done, a systematic mediastinal lymph node dissection was also carried out regardless of the gross appearance of the lymph nodes [4]. A postsurgical or pathologic stage was then obtained and recorded after histologic review of all removed specimens. The term "pathologic stage I" was reserved for patients with confirmed absence of mediastinal node metastases after careful microscopic examination of all excised material. As per criteria of the AJC, stage I carcinoma included the following groups of cancers: T1N0M0, T1N1M0, T2N0M0, and TisN0M0 (carcinoma in situ).

Sixty-five of the 169 lung cancers found (38%) had clinical stage I disease at the time of diagnosis. Sixty-two were classified stage I after thoracotomy and resection. Fifty-five had lobectomy and seven had wedge resection because limited pulmonary reserve precluded more extensive surgery. Three of these were found to have tumor microscopically at the resection margin. All had mediastinal lymph node dissection with histologic examination that confirmed the mediastinum to be free of metastasis. Survival was calculated from the date of detection of their lung cancer. Fifty-four of the original 62 patients with stage I disease are now alive (87%). There was one

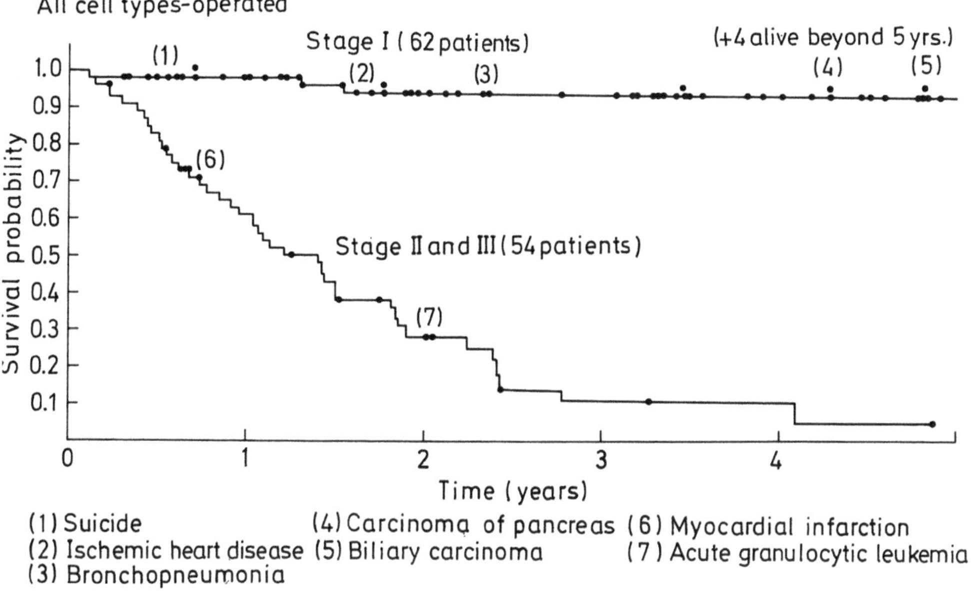

Fig. 1. Survival of patients operated for stage I and stage II or III lung cancer. Courtesy of Cancer [see Ref. 10]

postoperative death from a perforated esophagitis. Five died of unrelated causes without residual carcinoma, three died of distant metastases. There were three patients with stage I disease who were poor candidates for surgical treatment and were hence not operated. One has since died at 28 months, and two are alive with disease at 27 and 35 months respectively.

The remaining 104 men had stage II or III disease at the time of detection. Fifty-four were operated and their tumor resected. Forty of these have since died of their lung cancer after a median survival of 12 months. Two died of other causes and 12 are alive. Of the 50 men with advanced disease considered unresectable, 47 have died of their lung cancer. Only three are alive. Thus, only 15 of 104 with stage II or III lung cancer are presently alive, and only five of these have survived longer than 2 years.

The survival of patients with stage I disease treated surgically was compared with the survival of the patients with stage II or III disease also treated surgically (Fig. 1). Survival curves were calculated according to the Kaplan-Meier method. The 5-year survival for patients with resected stage I lung cancer is calculated to be 90%.

In the population screened, the distribution of lung cancer by cell type was almost exactly the same for stage I as for stages II and III, except in the case of oat cell carcinoma, which had an overwhelming preponderance of advanced stages. On our initial examination of the screenees (prevalence) we found only one oat cell carcinoma in 55 men with lung cancer. In subsequent examinations (incidence), oat cell carcinoma comprised 25% of all lung cancers.

There have been 40 interval cases of lung carcinoma, that is, cases diagnosed between screening examinations because of symptoms or because of chest X-rays taken for other reasons. Eighteen of the 40 were oat cell carcinomas, and only two of the 40 were stage I lung cancers at the time of diagnosis. The screening procedure used by us was not successful in detecting oat cell carcinoma early; only two of 27 were found in stage I. However, 45% of all non-oat cell carcinomas were detected in stage I and, interestingly, by the third year in the study, 60% of all newly developing non-oat cell carcinomas were detected in stage I. This may be attributable to more accurate chest X-ray interpretation, which is possible when previous annual X-rays are compared and minimal changes detected.

The relative value of sputum cytology and chest X-ray for detection of early cancer differs in the initial (prevalence) and subsequent (incidence) examinations. On the initial examination, approximately equal numbers of stage I lung carcinoma were detected by both techniques. On subsequent examinations, there were approximately five new lung carcinomas in stage I detected by chest X-ray for each one found by sputum cytology. It is important to note that the stage I cancers detected by cytology were epidermoid carcinomas of major bronchi, while those detected by X-ray were peripheral and about two-thirds were adenocarcinomas; only one of the 65 cases was detected simultaneously by both techniques. The greater number of early, radiologically occult epidermoid carcinomas detected by sputum cytology on initial (prevalence) examination compared with subsequent (incidence) examinations is consistent with a prolonged, slowly developing phase of the disease at this early stage.

The effect of screening on lung cancer mortality can be estimated only indirectly at this time. However, we have shown that close to 40% of all lung cancers can be detected early, in stage I, by present radiologic and cytologic screening techniques, and more than 90% of those detected in that favorable stage, and resected, can be expected to remain free of lung cancer for 5 years.

Some increase in survival time of patients with early stage lung cancer may be deceptive, due to what has been called "lead time". That is, earlier diagnosis in an asymptomatic phase will necessarily increase the time from detection to death even though there may be no actual prolongation of life. It is particularly difficult to evaluate lead time if early detection and treatment is thought to prolong life but does not cure. Unfortunately, there is no data on the clinical course of untreated stage I lung cancer. Until all patients in this study are followed to death, either from their lung cancer or some other cause, there is always the possibility that those who are treated for stage I lung cancer and appear to be cured clinically may yet develop recurrent or metastatic tumor and die of the disease.

If the treatment of lung cancer is of any value in prolonging survival and also in reducing mortality, it is likely to be more effective when the tumor burden is small and the individual is still healthy − that means early detection, early diagnosis, and early treatment. There are, as yet, no specific tumor markers in lung carcinoma to help detect this disease at an early stage or detect its recurrence after treatment. Only two methods are available for the detection of lung cancer: chest X-ray and sputum cytology. Whereas X-ray can detect small peripheral carcinomas that may be early, the early central lesions are not generally X-ray visible and can only be detected on sputum cytology. Yet not all cancers detected in this manner are necessarily early cancer. Some are late, despite detection at an asymptomatic stage. Not until the workup is complete and the tumor is removed can one state with confidence that an early carcinoma was present.

In the X-ray occult tumors, detection depends on sputum cytology, but localization depends on careful bronchoscopic evaluation of the tracheobronchial tree. The presence of cancer cells in sputum does not necessarily imply that a tumor is in the lung or bronchus as opposed to the upper airways, nor does it imply an early carcinoma. Nearly 30% of positive sputa from radiologically occult lesions in the New York program have come from cancers of head and neck origin.

Occult carcinomas of the lung represent a very small group of lung cancers. They make up less than one half of 1% of all lung cancers seen. Although the numbers are small, there is evidence that early removal of these tumors after detection and localization may result in an improved cancer cure rate and not simply be a gain in lead time. In an attempt to answer this question, we elected to combine our Memorial experience with that of the National Lung Program. From 1947 to present, 54 occult lung carcinomas were seen in 47 patients [6]. Seven had two separate occult lung carcinomas. In 1974 we reported 26 patients with occult carcinoma [7]. The majority of these had hemoptysis. Since our participation in a national early lung cancer detection program most of our occult carcinomas have been detected at an asymptomatic stage.

As fiberoptic bronchoscopy was not available until the late sixties, localization by rigid bronchoscopy was limited to central lesions. Bronchograms were necessary to identify the more peripheral lesions, and in some instances, exploratory thoracotomy was performed with what is now considered to be inadequate evidence of localization, with negative findings. Since the advent of the fiberoptic bronchoscope, localization by fiberoptic bronchoscopy has been possible in virtually every instance. Bronchograms have not been necessary. Of the recently reviewed tumors, 80% have been peripheral in location and not thoracotomy has been performed without precise localization of the tumor.

Although all patients seen presented with X-ray occult carcinomas, their stage of disease at presentation was variable. Thirty-three had stage I disease and 14 had stage II or III disease. We have defined early carcinomas to be tumors classified as stage I at treatment and advanced carcinomas as stage II or III at treatment, in accordance with the AJC staging.

From the early series of 26 patients reported in 1974, 13, or one half, had either advanced disease at treatment or early disease treated by nonsurgical means. All 13 have since died of their tumor, with a median survival of 15 months.

The remaining 13 of the 26 patients, i.e., the other half, had their tumors localized and treated by resection while still at an early stage. Their average survival has now reached 9 years and the median survival is 8 years. Five are still alive and well 8−20 years later. One is alive at 9 years with a second lung carcinoma and six have died of other causes 2−17 years later.

An additional 21 patients with occult carcinoma were seen and treated since the last report, and 14, or two thirds of these, also had early tumors at treatment, five being pure in situ carcinomas. The median survival to date in this group of patients is 46 months, but follow-up is still short. Thirteen of the 14 are now alive, 11 free of disease, and two with new carcinomas, one in the lung and one of the biliary tree. One patient died of carcinoma of the pancreas at 50 months. An additional patient with clinical stage I disease had severe emphysema precluding surgical resection. He has an epidermoid carcinoma in the subsegmental bronchus, believed to be in situ or focally invasive, and was treated by endoscopic electrocoagulation. He is now alive with persistent disease at 33 months, and his chest X-ray is still normal.

Of a total of 27 patients with early lung cancer treated by resection since 1949 to the present, none has had recurrence of his original tumor after follow-up extending from 12 months to 20 years. They are either alive and well or have since died of other causes.

Because of an anticipated long survival, patients with occult carcinomas remain at risk to develop second cancers, usually a second airway carcinoma. Two separate cancers were identified in 21 of the 47 patients (45%). Fifteen (32%) had a second lung cancer, seven of which were second occult carcinomas. The interval between two carcinomas varied from a synchronous presentation to 30 years, with a median interval of $3^1/_2$ years.

It is significant that only patients with early disease treated by excision have done well and lived for long periods of time. In contrast, patients with presumed early disease treated by other means have done poorly.

Peripheral carcinomas detected on routine chest X-rays are frequently early cancers. In our recent experience at Memorial Hospital, nearly 30% of all lung cancers seen had stage I disease. We had demonstrated in an earlier report that the 1-, 2-, and 3-year survival after resection in this group of patients was 93%, 87%, and 85% respectively [5]. We have since been able to obtain further follow-up on these patients and the 5-year survival is now calculated to be nearly 70% without correction for operative mortality or deaths from other causes. The need is clearly to diagnose and treat more lung cancers at an early, asymptomatic stage.

References

1. Flehinger BJ, Smart, JS (1978) Computer simulation of a screening program for the early detection of cancer. IBM Thomas/Watson Research Center, Rye, New York
2. Flehinger BJ, Melamed MR, Heelan RT, McGinnis CM, Zaman MB, Martini N (1978) Accuracy of chest film screening for technologists in the New York early lung cancer detection program. Am J Roentgenol 131: 593−597
3. Heelan RT, Melamed MR, Zaman MB, Marini N, Flehinger BJ (to be published) X-ray diagnosis of oat cell cancer in a higher risk screened population. Radiology
4. Martini N (1976) Improved methods of recording data in lung cancer. Clin Bull (Mem Sloan-Kettering Cancer Cent) 6: 93−98
5. Martini N, Beattie EJ Jr (1977) Results of surgical treatment in stage I lung cancer. J Thorac Cardiovasc Surg 74: 499−505
6. Martini N, Melamed MR (to be published) Occult carcinomas of the lung. Ann Thorac Surg
7. Martini N, Beattie EJ Jr, Cliffton EE, Melamed MR (1974) Radiologically occult lung cancer: report of 26 cases. Surg Clin North Am 54: 811−823
8. Melamed MR, Flehinger BJ, Miller D et al. (1977a) Preliminary report of the lung cancer detection program in New York. Cancer 39: 369−382
9. Melamed MR, Zaman MB, Flehinger BJ, Martini N (1977b) Radiologically occult in situ and incipient invasive epidermoid lung cancer. Am J Surg Pathol 1: 5−16
10. Melamed MR, Flehinger BJ, Zaman MB, Heelan RT, Hallerman ET, Martini N (to be published) Detection of true pathologic stage I lung cancer in a screening program and the effects on survival. Cancer
11. National Cancer Institute Cooperative Early Lung Cancer Group (1979) Revised manual of procedures. Natl Inst Health
12. American Joint Committee for Cancer Staging and End-Results Reporting, Task Force on Lung (1980) Staging of lung cancer 1979. Chicago

Results of the Mayo Lung Project: An Interim Report

D. Sanderson and R. Fontana

Mayo Clinic and Mayo Foundation, Division of Thoracic Diseases and Internal Medicine, Rochester, MN, USA

Recognizing the enormous increase of lung cancer as a public health problem, the National Cancer Institute initiated three large clinical trials of screening in the 1970s at the Mayo Clinic, Johns Hopkins, and Memorial Sloan-Kettering. The only available tests for identifying presymptomatic lung cancer are roentgenography of the chest and sputum cytology. These tests were given different emphases in the three studies, with the Mayo Lung Project (MLP) seeking to evaluate the effects of repeating chest roentgenography and sputum tests at 4-month intervals in a high risk population as compared with a similar control population not systematically rescreened [2]. The Memorial and Hopkins studies include frequent sputum cytology, but only annual chest roentgenography. The 4-month interval in the MLP was selected because earlier studies had suggested equivocal benefit at 6-month intervals, and 4 months seemed the most frequent with which even health-conscious subjects might be expected to comply.

Random screening of the general population was not intended, inasmuch as lung cancer is not randomly distributed. Among several possible risk factors, the MLP sought to concentrate on three: sex, age, and smoking habits. Subjects were selected from patients coming to the Mayo Clinic for physical examinations. All men older than age 45 years were given a questionnaire about smoking. Those who smoked more than 20 cigarettes daily or had done so within the preceding year were sent to the MLP office for an interview. The interview confirmed the age and smoking habits and sought to exclude those with a prior history of tumor of the respiratory tract. All men had initial cytology of a 3-day pooled sputum sample and chest roentgenography (14×17 inch posteroanterior X-ray view). Sputum cytology samples were processed by the Saccomanno technique and screened initially by cytotechnologists. All abnormal samples and randomly selected normal specimens were analyzed by the same cytopathologist. All chest X-ray films were interpreted intially by a staff radiologist and then reviewed by two MLP physicians, either two radiologists or one radiologist and one pulmonary physician. Abnormal findings were investigated, and these data constituted our prevalence screening cases.

Subjects with no evidence of lung cancer on initial screening were randomized to either the close surveillance group, in which tests were to be repeated every 4 months, or the control group, for which annual tests were *advised*.

Participants in the 4-monthly screening tests who lived remote from Rochester, Minnesota, mailed sputum jars to our laboratory and also serial chest roentgenograms.

Recent Results in Cancer Research, Vol. 82
© Springer-Verlag Berlin · Heidelberg 1982

All films again had dual readings, as well as comparison with the initial chest roentgenogram. If interpretations differed, a third physician refereed. Findings that were suggestive of lung cancer were followed by one of the MLP clinicians. When circumstances permitted, the patients returned to Rochester, Minnesota, for further investigation and treatment. If distance or other factors prevented that return, communication about treatment was maintained with the patients's home medical advisor.

Patients in the control population were contacted by letter annually to determine state of health, any interval illness or treatment, and smoking habits. Although all patients had been advised initially to seek annual testing, few actually followed that advice.

Follow-up of all patients has been excellent, less than 1% of both groups having been lost.

Results of Prevalence Screen

Of 11,001 men originally interviewed, 63 were ineligible because of prior respiratory tract cancer or presence of lung cancer at their initial visit. Thus 10,938 entered the prevalence screening, and lung cancer was found in 92 (or 8.4 per 1,000). Age-specific prevalence increased with each 5-year increment (Table 1).

Roentgenography was the most frequent means of detection of lung cancer, accounting for 59 cases. Sixteen cases were detected by sputum cytology, and 17 were identified by both (Table 2). "Curative" resection was the most frequent for those with

Table 1. Age-specific prevalence of lung cancer

Age (years)	Screened (No.)	Lung cancer cases (No.)	Prevalence rate (per 1,000 screened)
45–49	2,644	3	1.1
50–54	2,613	17	6.5
55–59	2,479	24	9.7
60–64	1,913	26	13.6
≥65	1,298	22	17.1
All ages	10,938	92	8.4

Table 2. Prevalence cases of lung cancer: Method of detection

Method of detection	Cases (No.)	"Curative" resection (No.)	%
Roentgenography	59	30	51
Cytology	16	15	94
Both	17	5	29
Total	92	50	54

Table 3. Prevalence cases of lung cancer: Cell type

Cell type	Cases (No.)	"Curative" resection	
		(No.)	%
Squamous	40	31	78
Adenocarcinoma	24	8	33
Large cell	16	11	69
Small cell	12	0	0
Total	92	50	54

Table 4. Prevalence cases of lung cancer: AJC stage

Stage	Cases	
	No.	% of total
I Postsurgical	39	42
Clinical	4	4
II	7	8
III	42	46
Total	92	100

"occult" cancer, however, and less common when both cytologic and X-ray findings were abnormal. All cell types were represented, but squamous cell cancer was most frequent, found in 40 of the 92 cases. Small cell undifferentiated cancer was present in 12 (13%), as shown in Table 3.

All patients were staged by the criteria of the American Joint Committee for Cancer Staging and End-Results Reporting (AJC), and almost half had stage I cancer (Table 4).

Incidence Screening

After the initial screening to exclude patients with cancer of the respiratory tract, records were reviewed to exclude also those with other serious medical problems that made participation in a continued screening program impractical. Likewise omitted from the prospective screening were those who refused or failed to complete the initial sputum test, roentgenography, or both. The remaining group consisted of 4,624 participants having 4-monthly tests and 4,598 controls, a total of 9,222 subjects. Analysis of characteristics of the two groups showed no significant difference in age, smoking habits, exposure to other pollutants or carcinogens, and history of chronic bronchitis.

Through April 1, 1980, new cases of lung cancer (incidence cases) occurred in 110 of the 4-monthly surveillance patients and in 78 control subjects. Incidence rates were greater for the 4-monthly participants (4.7 per 1,000 per year) than for the control subjects (3.4 per 1,000 per year). Moreover, incidence rates for each cell type were

Table 5. Incidence cases of lung cancer: comparison of incidence rates in 4-monthly surveillance and control groups

	4-monthly			Control		
	No.	Cases % of total	Incidence rate (per 1,000 per year)	No.	Cases % of total	Incidence rate (per 1,000 per year)
Total	110	100.0	4.7	78	100.0	3.4
Postsurgical stage I	51	46.3	2.2	16	20.5	0.7
All other stages	58	52.7	2.5	61	78.2	2.6
Squamous	32	29.1	1.4	26	33.3	1.1
Adenocarcinoma	26	23.6	1.1	19	24.4	0.8
Large cell	20	18.2	0.8	10	12.8	0.4
Small cell	28	25.5	1.2	22	28.2	1.0
Non-small cell	81	73.6	3.4	55	70.5	2.4

Because of incomplete data, one of the 100 four-monthly incidence cases and one of the 78 control incidence cases have been excluded from the analysis by stage and cell type. In three close surveillance cases, cell type is unknown

Table 6. Incidence of lung cancer: age at detection

Groups	Age at detection (years)					Total
	45−49	50−54	55−59	60−64	≥ 65	
4-Monthly						
Cases (no.)	2	11	20	23	54	110
Person-years	2,774.2	5,810.8	5,583.1	4,828.0	4,486.9	23,482.9
Rate (per 1,000 per year)	0.7	1.9	3.6	4.8	12.0	4.7
Control						
Cases (no.)	2	6	11	26	33	78
Person-years	2,745.4	5,723.3	5,525.6	4,594.7	4,447.6	23,036.6
Rate (per 1,000 per year)	0.7	1.0	2.0	5.7	7.4	3.4

greater among the participants than among the controls (Table 5). More than three times as many postsurgical stage I cases of lung cancer were identified by screening than were found in the control group.

As with the initial prevalence screening, age was an important determinant of incidence of lung cancer. Incidence rates were less than 1 per 1,000 per year in patients younger than age 50 years, and increased with each 5-year increment (Table 6). Chest X-ray films were the most frequent means of detection of incidence cases of lung cancer (Table 7). Some patients sought medical care in their home communities, at which time nonstudy X-ray films disclosed abnormalities that led to the diagnosis.

Table 7. Incidence cases of lung cancer: method of detection

Method of detection	4-monthly			Control		
	No.	"Curative" resection		No.	"Curative" resection	
		(No.)	%		(No.)	%
Study roentgenography	53	34	64	–	–	–
Cytology	12	11	92	–	–	–
Both of the above	6	5	83	–	–	–
Nonstudy roentgenography	16	8	50	26	14	54
Symptoms	20	3	15	51	7	14
Autopsy	2	–	–	0	0	0
Total	109	61	56	77	21	27

Because of incomplete data, one of the 110 four-monthly incidence cases and one of the 78 control incidence cases have been excluded from the analysis

Table 8. Incidence cases of lung cancer: cell type

Cell type	4-monthly			Control		
	No.	"Curative" resection		No.	"Curative" resection	
		(No.)	%		(No.)	%
Squamous	32	27	84	26	10	38
Adenocarcinoma	26	16	62	19	7	37
Large cell	20	12	60	10	3	30
Small cell	28	5	18	22	1	5
Other, unknown	3	1	33	–	–	–
Total	109	61	56	77	21	27

Because of incomplete data, one of the 110 four-monthly incidence cases and one of the 78 control incidence cases have been excluded from the analysis

Symptoms of lung cancer prompted patients to seek medical attention and led to the diagnosis in more than $2\,^1/_2$ times as many control subjects as participants.

Histologic types among the incidence cases of lung cancer varied somewhat from those found in the initial prevalence cases. Although squamous cell cancer still predominated, 26% of the 4-monthly screened participants and 29% of the control subjects had small cell undifferentiated cancers (Table 8). Resectability was almost three times greater in the close surveillance group than in the control group, primarily because of the more favorable stage of cancer in patients with squamous and large cell carcinoma and adenocarcinoma.

There were 51 patients with postsurgical stage I cancers among the participants, as compared with 16 among the controls. The relatively high number of stage III cases in both groups resulted from the high incidence of small cell cancers (Table 9).

Because of lead time and length bias, caution is necessary in examining survival results after treatment of lung cancer. But unless early treatment has some effect on survival

Table 9. Incidence cases of lung cancer: AJC stage

Stage	4-Monthly		Control	
	No.	%	No.	%
I Postsurgical	51	47	16	21
Clinical	9[a]	8	5	6
II	3	3	3	4
III	46	42	53	69
Total	109	100	77	100

Because of incomplete data, one of the 110 four-monthly incidence cases and one of the 78 control incidence cases have been excluded from the analysis

[a] Includes one squamous cell stage I case detected by sputum cytology, but proved at autopsy after the subject had died from other causes

Probability of surviving (%)

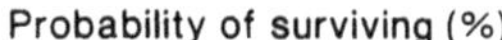
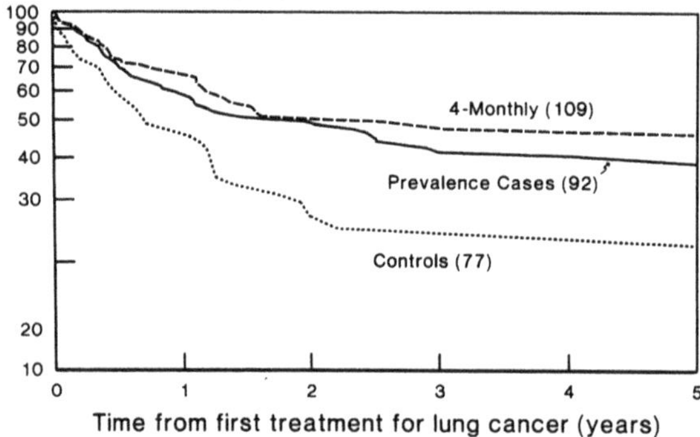

Fig. 1. Survival curves for patients in both prevalence and incidence lung cancer groups

Probability of Surviving (%)

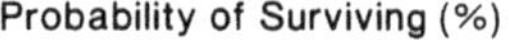
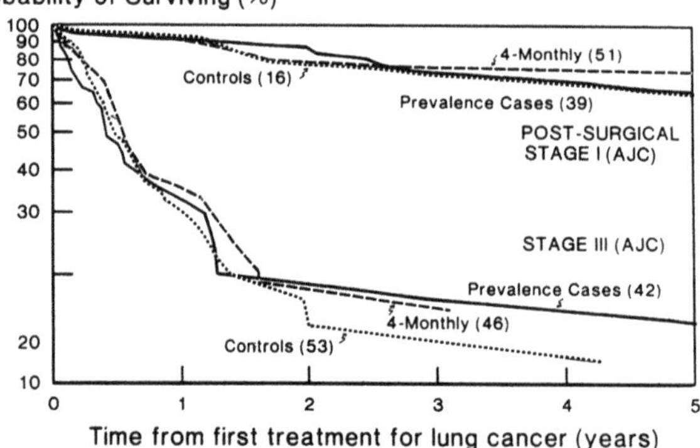

Fig. 2. Survival curves for patients in both prevalence and incidence lung cancer groups by stages

curves, it is impossible to find changes in mortality rates. Figure 1 shows survival curves for patients in both prevalence and incidence lung cancer groups. Figure 2 demonstrates the effects of staging in both groups; the greatest benefit from earlier detection seems to be the identification of more patients with the more favorable stage I category of cancer.

Table 10. Incidence cases of lung cancer: comparison of death rates in 4-monthly surveillance and control groups

	4-Monthly		Control	
	Deaths (No.)	Death rate (per 1,000 per year)	Deaths (No.)	Death rate (per 1,000 per year)
Total	51	2.2	54	2.3
Postsurgical stage I	11	0.5	5	0.2
All other stages	40	1.7	49	2.1
Squamous	9	0.4	16	0.7
Adenocarcinoma	8	0.3	12	0.5
Large cell	11	0.5	7	0.3
Small cell	21	0.9	19	0.8
Unknown	2	0.1	0	0.0
Non-small cell	30	1.3	35	1.5

There were 39% fewer deaths in the screened group from squamous cell and adenocarcinoma than in the control group (17 versus 28); on the other hand, there seemed to be no reduction in deaths from undifferentiated carcinomas (Table 10).

Discussion

It is evident now that a screening program with chest roentgenography and sputum cytology can be conducted in a defined high risk group. Most persons who leave the screening program do so within the first year, and overall compliance with continued testing approximates 80%.

The screening program does detect lung cancer at earlier stages, when surgical resection can be accomplished more effectively. Unfortunately, the incidence of rapidly growing small cell undifferentiated lung cancer is high in this population, and these patients seem to benefit minimally by early detection.

Localization of occult cancers detected by sputum cytology has been thought to be difficult. In our experience and that of the other cooperative early lung cancer groups, however, localization has been consistently possible [1]. These patients have had more resectable and more limited disease than other patients.

The difference in number of cases of cancer identified in the control population and the 4-monthly surveillance group remains an enigma. The two groups were almost identical in most respects, including age, smoking habits, occupational exposures, cessation of smoking after entering the study, and deaths from other causes.

Because control subjects were contacted by mail only annually, there was a delay in learning about changes in their health. This delay factor should be eliminated with longer follow-up or by backdating analysis of results, but thus far we have seen no trend to equalize these incidence rates by these measures. Another concern is the unrecognized incidence cases of lung cancer in the control population. In these patients, death might be ascribed to other conditions. Nevertheless, we have not seen excess deaths from other pulmonary causes, such as pneumonia, either on death certificates or in other "best information" sources.

Summary

Screening for lung cancer by chest roentgenography and sputum cytology can be conducted by mail. Detection, localization, and treatment of early presymptomatic lesions are possible. The initial prevalence of lung cancer in men older than age 45 years who were heavy smokers was almost 1%. Rescreening at 4-monthly intervals detected 4.7 new cases of lung cancer per 1,000 subjects per year. Three times as many postsurgical stage I lesions were detected in the screened group as in the control group. Although survival seems to have been improved by screening, mortality from lung cancer is not yet significantly different in the 4-monthly surveillance and control groups. Longer follow-up is necessary for determination of the ultimate usefulness of screening.

References

1. Sanderson DR, Fontana RS (1975) Early lung cancer detection and localization. Ann Otol Rhinol Laryngol 84: 583–588
2. Taylor WF, Fontana RS (1972) Biometric design of the Mayo lung project for early detection and localization of lung cancer. Cancer 30: 1344–1347

Subject Index

Recent Results in Cancer Research

Sponsored by the Swiss League against Cancer. Editor in Chief: P. Rentchnick, Genève

GPSR Compliance
The European Union's (EU) General Product Safety Regulation (GPSR) is a set
of rules that requires consumer products to be safe and our obligations to
ensure this.

If you have any concerns about our products, you can contact us on

ProductSafety@springernature.com

In case Publisher is established outside the EU, the EU authorized
representative is:

Springer Nature Customer Service Center GmbH
Europaplatz 3
69115 Heidelberg, Germany

www.ingramcontent.com/pod-product-compliance
Ingram Content Group UK Ltd.
Pitfield, Milton Keynes, MK11 3LW, UK
UKHW052347070726
473059UK00009B/2584